THE LOW-CARB
DIABETES
SOLUTION
COOKBOOK

DANA CARPENDER

THE LOW-CARB

DIABETES

SOLUTION

COOKBOOK

Prevent and Heal Type 2 Diabetes
with 200 Ultra Low-Carb Recipes

FAIR WINDS

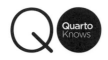

Quarto is the authority on a wide range of topics.

Quarto educates, entertains and enriches the lives of
our readers—enthusiasts and lovers of hands-on living.

www.QuartoKnows.com

First published in the United States of America in 2016 by
Fair Winds Press, an imprint of Quarto Publishing Group USA Inc.
100 Cummings Center, Suite 406-L, Beverly, Massachusetts 01915-6101
Telephone: (978) 282-9590, Fax: (978) 283-2742
QuartoKnows.com
Visit our blogs at QuartoKnows.com

20 19 18 17 16   1 2 3 4 5

ISBN: 978-1-59233-729-3

Digital edition published in 2016
eISBN: 978-1-63159-173-0

Library of Congress Cataloging-in-Publication Data available

Design and Page Layout: Laura H. Couallier, Laura Herrmann Design

Printed in the United States of America

*The information in this book is for educational purposes only. It is not intended to replace the advice of a physician
or medical practitioner. Please see your health-care provider before beginning any new health program.*

CONTENTS

FOREWORD

It is my great pleasure to write this foreword for The Low-Carb Diabetes Solution Cookbook, by Dana Carpender. This book is a fundamental part of the HEAL Diabetes & Medical Weight Loss Clinics program, and will make the transition to an LCHF (low-carbohydrate, high-fat) lifestyle seem effortless! HEAL stands for "Healthier Eating and Living," and the HEAL Protocol integrates medical, dietary, psychological, and fitness interventions delivered at HEAL clinics and remotely, 24/7, using digital health and tele- medicine tools.

As director of the Duke Lifestyle Medicine Clinic since 2007, I have used the dietary basis of the HEAL Protocol as a natural extension of the research that had been done at Duke University and other research centers around the world. My interest in LCHF began while I was an internal medicine specialist: Two of my patients used LCHF (Atkins Induction Diet) to lose weight in 1998. It clearly worked, but I was skeptical and concerned about the safety because of all the fat in the diet. But if it were safe, I knew that this could be an important lifestyle tool to treat obesity and diabetes. The research since that time has demonstrated the safety of this approach.

The past few years have shown a large shift in attitudes toward LCHF lifestyles. A 2014 Time magazine story, with the cover line "Eat Butter. Scientists labeled fat the enemy. Why they were wrong," helped advance the popularization of LCHF into mainstream U.S. culture. Additional research studies have been published that confirm the positive effects of LCHF lifestyles on diabetes; LCHF continues to be popular in Sweden (www.dietdoctor.com); and the first Low Carb Health Summit was held in February 2015 in Cape Town, South Africa. (Lectures are available for viewing at www.lchfconvention.com.) South Africa has become aware of LCHF through Professor Timothy Noakes, an exercise guru who changed his advice for athletes away from "carb loading" and toward carbohydrate restriction before athletic competition. More and more athletes are turning to LCHF for the benefits in their performance.

Despite the research, the most common concern that people have about the low-carbohydrate lifestyle is: "But what will happen to my blood cholesterol level by eating all that fat?" A whole generation of doctors, dietitians, and the general public was taught that eating fat and cholesterol would raise "bad" LDL blood cholesterol and cause heart disease. This "diet-heart hypothesis" was the theory that spawned the low-fat diet fad. I was privileged to be a part of the studies about the LCHF diet, and the predictions about how the LCHF diets would worsen the blood lipid profile didn't come true when they were actually studied. It turned out that the LCHF diet reduced health risks by lowering blood triglycerides and raising the "good" HDL cholesterol. At the time of publication, the revised 2015 USDA/NIH Dietary Guidelines for Americans are poised to take away the limitations on dietary fat and cholesterol.

At the HEAL clinics, the LCHF diet is used as a therapeutic tool to turn around and fix most of the chronic medical conditions that are seen today. But LCHF is also a healthy diet that prevents these same chronic medical conditions. LCHF is an excellent treatment for diabetes, high blood pressure, gastroesophageal reflux disorder, high blood triglycerides, low blood HDL cholesterol, polycystic ovarian syndrome, and irritable bowel disease. Often the improvement that we see is "unbelievable"—meaning that other doctors and experts don't believe it. Weight loss of 200 pounds (more than 90 kg), lowering of blood triglycerides by 900 mg/dL (10.2 mmol/L), increasing the "good" HDL cholesterol by 50 mg/dL (1.3 mmol/L)—doctors often are in disbelief, and because the studies haven't been published, the researchers say the evidence "doesn't exist." However, these are the clinical outcomes that we observe.

I'm excited to be a part of the HEAL Diabetes & Medical Weight Loss Clinics for those who need medical supervision during the treatment of diabetes and obesity. I am confident that this cookbook will be a great resource for you as you follow the HEAL Protocol.

—Eric C. Westman, M.D., M.H.S.
HEAL Diabetes & Medical Weight Loss Clinics

Eric C. Westman is board certified in Internal Medicine and Obesity Medicine, with a master's degree in Clinical Research from Duke University and over 90 peer-reviewed publications on his clinical research regarding treatments for obesity, diabetes, and tobacco dependence. He is a Co-Founder of HEAL Diabetes & Medical Weight Loss Clinics, Director of the Duke Lifestyle Medicine Clinic, Past President of the Obesity Medicine Association, and is a Fellow of both The Obesity Society and the Obesity Medicine Association.

FOREWORD

If you have type 2 diabetes and are also overweight, you are faced with two chronic conditions. To be successful in managing your health, you need to make changes in the way you eat for a lifetime. If you don't stay in control with the proper lifestyle changes, both of these conditions will get worse over time. To help you succeed, you need knowledge and the proper tools.

The HEAL Protocol will give you the knowledge to help you understand how and why controlling both the quality and the quantity of carbohydrate foods can be so effective in putting diabetes into remission and losing those excess pounds. This cookbook is one of the tools that can keep you on track by providing easy-to-make, fun, nourishing, and tasty meals.

Even if you don't cook, Dana Carpender will help you make your way around the kitchen. Eating out regularly can sabotage your weight loss efforts. If you have diabetes, it isn't likely you will achieve the best level of success by always eating out. Cooking whole foods does not have to be difficult or overwhelming.

At first, changing your food choices may seem difficult. But in my view, not making those changes and suffering the consequences is more devastating. This cookbook is targeted especially to people with diabetes who are serious about controlling their weight and blood sugar levels without the use of potentially dangerous and expensive medications. It can be done. People do it all the time.

One surefire way to succeed is to ride the coattails of someone who has been successful. Do what they do. Dana has twenty years of personal experience living a low-carb lifestyle. I have been on low carb since 1974. I have a family history of type 2 diabetes on my father's side and morbid obesity on my mother's. As a nurse, I knew I had to be proactive if I was going to avoid these conditions. So far I have been very successful at avoiding diabetes and managing my weight comfortably without hunger.

Dana and I both know the pitfalls that can lead to failure in the long run. Major stumbling blocks include boredom with meals, facing hunger with no good food choices, or having to count calories. This book will offer you a wide range of ideas while keeping your carb intake at no more than 5 grams per meal.

I have enjoyed Dana's other cookbooks, which increased my menu choices, and look forward to more ideas in this one.

—Jacqueline A. Eberstein, R.N.

Jacqueline A. Eberstein is one of the foremost authorities on the Atkins Lifestyle. In 1974 she began working with Dr. Robert Atkins as the Head Nurse in his weight-loss clinic. She later became the Director of Medical Education at The Atkins Center for Complementary Medicine, in New York City. After The Atkins Center closed in 2003, she became the Director of Nutrition Information for Atkins Health and Medical Information Services. While there she co-authored Atkins Diabetes Revolution. She is currently the Director of Protocol for HEAL.

This book is dedicated to all the doctors, nurses, dietitians, and other health professionals who have had the courage to confront the fact that everything they'd been told about nutrition was wrong—that the low-fat diet they'd been recommending was hurting, not helping, people—and change course in the face of scorn and opposition. You are heroes.

CHAPTER 1

Diabetes: The Problem and How to Solve It

Welcome to this book, and to the HEAL family. We're sorry that your health has driven you to search for a solution, but we're glad to have you with us. You're in the right place.

HEAL Diabetes & Medical Weight Loss Clinics have a simple mission: to teach "Healthier Eating and Living," and by doing so, restore people to health. Eric C. Westman, M.D., M.H.S., our founder and president, and Jacqueline A. Eberstein, R.N., a medical advisor, have, between them, taught thousands of people with diabetes to not merely control the progression of their disease, but to put it into total remission.

Me? I write low-carbohydrate cookbooks. I have eaten a low-carbohydrate diet for twenty years now. I was never diagnosed with diabetes, but have had a doctor, looking at my charts, say that I would surely be diabetic by now had I not changed my diet in 1995.

I know Dr. Westman and Jackie Eberstein because of my longtime involvement with the low-carb community. When Dr. Westman told me he was starting a chain of diabetes treatment centers, with the goal of teaching people to eat a low-carbohydrate diet, I knew I had to be involved. They deal with the medical part and have vetted everything I say here. I'm the one who can help you figure out the question "What do I eat now?" I promise, the answer to that question is varied, delicious, and satisfying.

WHAT IS DIABETES?

There are two kinds of diabetes. They both involve problems with insulin, the hormone that ushers sugar out of the bloodstream and into the cells, and lead to high blood sugar. However, the causes of the problem are quite different.

Type 1, or juvenile-onset diabetes, is due to failure of the insulin-secreting beta cells in the pancreas. People with type 1 diabetes simply lack insulin. According to the American Diabetes Association (ADA) website, only 5 percent of people with diabetes have this form of the disease.

In type 2 diabetes, the pancreas makes insulin, but the insulin receptors, or the "doors" on the cells that insulin should open, are not working properly to move sugar out of the bloodstream, a condition called insulin resistance. Blood sugar levels start rising. The beta cells secrete more and more insulin, trying to force the faulty insulin receptors to respond. Eventually, the beta cells start to fail, producing less and less insulin, and blood sugar rises inexorably.

It is type 2 diabetes that has been increasing at a frightening rate all over the world.

THE MODERN EPIDEMIC

The numbers are staggering. According to the Centers for Disease Control and Prevention (CDC), more than 29 million people in the United States are affected by diabetes, with one in four of those cases as yet undiagnosed. Another 86 million Americans —one in three adults—have pre-diabetes and are on their way to full-blown diabetes. Without intervention, somewhere between 15 and 30 percent of people with prediabetes will develop diabetes within five years. The CDC estimates that one in three Americans will develop diabetes at some point.

What does this mean for the lives of these people?

- The National Institutes of Health (NIH) states that 60 to 70 percent of those with diabetes eventually suffer diabetic neuropathy, a degenerative condition of the nerves that causes numbness, tingling, and/or pain in the extremities. It can also cause muscle wasting, indigestion, nausea, vomiting, diarrhea, constipation, dizziness on standing, problems with urination, and erectile dysfunction.

- The American Podiatric Medical Association estimates that between 15 and 24 percent of people with diabetes develop ulcerated wounds on their feet.

- Diabetes is a major cause of amputations, often due to those ulcerated wounds. According to the CDC's *2014 National Diabetes Statistics Report*, seventy-three thousand people with diabetes had a limb amputated in 2010. Sixty percent of amputations in people over age twenty are due to diabetes.

- According to the National Eye Institute, 40 to 45 percent of those with diabetes develop diabetic retinopathy, the most common cause of new blindness in adults. The condition doubles the average person's risk of glaucoma and increases the risk of cataracts even more dramatically (two to five times the usual).

- The CDC's report also states that in 2011, because of diabetes, nearly fifty thousand people began treatment for kidney failure and more than a quarter of a million were living on dialysis or with a kidney transplant.

- Seventy-one percent of people with diabetes over the age of twenty-one have high blood pressure. People with diabetes have nearly double the risk of heart attack and one-and-a-half times the risk of stroke as those who do not have the disease.

- Diabetes increases susceptibility to other illnesses and can worsen their prognoses. For example, the CDC tells us that people with diabetes are more likely to die from pneumonia or influenza than people who do not have diabetes.

- The CDC's Diabetes Fact Sheet for 2011 tells us that people sixty or older with diabetes are two to three times more likely than those who do not have diabetes to report an inability to walk one-quarter of a mile, climb stairs, or do housework compared with people without diabetes in the same age group.

- The CDC also states that people with diabetes are twice as likely to have depression (which can complicate diabetes management) than people without diabetes. Interestingly, depression also appears to predispose sufferers to diabetes.

- According to the National Academy on an Aging Society, "The life expectancy of people with diabetes averages 15 years less than that of people without diabetes." That's nearly a 20 percent reduction in life span. The CDC concludes, "Overall, the risk for death among people with diabetes is about twice that of people of similar age but without diabetes."

Does this scare you? It should. Elevated blood sugar rots your body from the inside out, doing massive, global damage to both your body and your quality of life.

To add insult to genuine, crippling injury, diabetes threatens to bankrupt us. The rapidly escalating cost of medical care is among the greatest burdens facing the United States, and a frightening part of that cost is attributable to diabetes. In 2013, the journal *Diabetes Care* stated, "The total estimated cost of diagnosed diabetes in 2012 is $245 billion, including $176 billion in direct medical costs and $69 billion in reduced productivity."

What does that look like on an individual level? *Diabetes Care* breaks it down: "People with diagnosed diabetes incur average medical expenditures of about $13,700 per year, of which about $7,900 is attributed to diabetes. People with diagnosed diabetes, on average, have medical expenditures approximately 2.3 times higher than what expenditures would be in the absence of diabetes."

I'm sure you can think of more agreeable things to do with your money.

WHAT'S MAKING YOU SICK?

That diabetes is a disease of poor diet is not a new observation. Circa 600 BCE, the Indian physician Susruta said, "Madhumeha [honey urine] is a disease which the rich principally suffer from, and is brought on by their overindulgence in rice, flour and sugar."

Overindulgence was harder before modern agriculture, grocery stores, fast-food joints, convenience stores, and omnipresent soda machines. As indulgences of the rich became the staples of the middle class and then the impoverished, this disease of the affluent crossed cultural lines and is now ravaging the poor, who subsist on starches and sugar because they are cheap.

Yes, genetics appear to be involved as well; some people are more susceptible than others. But if genetics were the driving factor, diabetes would not have exploded, both here and worldwide. Genetics simply don't change that quickly. Diet has.

In 1977, led by Senator George McGovern, the federal government issued its first dietary guidelines, recommending that all Americans reduce fat —especially saturated fat—and cholesterol intake. Those guidelines also recommended an increase in starch intake. Suddenly, Americans "knew" that a healthy diet was based on grains, and that meat, butter, and eggs were the causes of heart disease.

We listened. According to the USDA's Economic Research Service, between 1970 and 1993, annual per capita grain consumption increased by an average of 54 pounds (24.5 kg), added sugars by 23 pounds (10.5 kg), fruit by 48 pounds (21.5 kg), and vegetables by a remarkable 61 pounds (27.5 kg). Simultaneously, egg consumption dropped by 76 per person per year, and milk consumption by 7 gallons (3.75 L) per year.

With low-fat, low-cholesterol diets being the new word in health, people with diabetes, at high risk of heart disease, were told to reduce fat and load up on "healthy whole grains."

Unfortunately, the saturated fat and cholesterol hypothesis of heart disease was wrong. In 2010, a meta-analysis appeared in the *American Journal of Clinical Nutrition*. It looked at twenty-one studies regarding the effects of saturated fat on heart disease and found "no significant evidence for concluding that dietary saturated fat is associated with an increased risk of CHD [coronary heart disease] or CVD [cardiovascular disease]."

Despite numerous articles debunking the dangers of saturated fat and cholesterol in the past decade—heck, the story made the cover of *Time* magazine in 2014—Americans are still being told to limit saturated fats and cholesterol and load up on starches. The USDA 2010 Dietary Guidelines for Americans recommend that adults get 45 to 65 percent of their calories from carbohydrates. Assuming a 2,000-calorie-per-day diet, that would be anywhere from 225 to 325 grams of carbohydrate per day. One hopes this will be amended in the guidelines due out by the end of 2015.

That's for ostensibly healthy people. What about diabetics, people with broken carbohydrate metabolisms? Unfortunately, many dietitians follow the old advice and recommend a carb-heavy diet for people with diabetes. Too many people trying to manage diabetes are still being told to eat carbs and use medication to "cover" the resultant blood sugar spikes.

Although the ADA has recently said that there is no one ideal diabetic diet, at the time of publication, the organization recommends starting at 45 to 60 grams of carbohydrate per meal. That's up to three times the carbohydrate we recommend in an entire day—and the ADA is also suggesting another 15 to 20 grams of carbohydrate in each snack. Whole grains appear among the group's list of "Diabetic Super Foods."

The ADA also continues to warn against saturated fats, saying, "To cut risk of heart disease and stroke, look at saturated and trans fats. Look for products with the lowest amount of saturated and trans fats per serving." (We agree with this advice about trans fats.)

The National Institutes of Health, at the time of publication, still recommends that people with diabetes eat six to ten servings of starches per day and two to four fruits, depending on body size and activity. The agency still recommends limiting meat and eggs to just 4 to 7 ounces (115 to 200 g) per day, and still shows the Food Pyramid, long since abandoned by the USDA, with the foundation still resting on starches. The NIH states: "Eat some starches at each meal. Eating starches is healthy for everyone, including people with diabetes." It does not elaborate.

The NIH recommendations lump fats in with sugars as foods to be carefully limited. What is said specifically about sweets? "Sweets can be high in carbohydrate and fat. Some contain saturated fats, trans fats, and cholesterol that increase your risk of heart disease." Saturated fats, not carbohydrates, are still the official bogeyman.

While pushing starches, the NIH recommends, "Eat fewer fried and high-fat starches such as regular tortilla chips and potato chips, french fries, pastries, or biscuits. Try pretzels, fat-free popcorn, baked tortilla chips or potato chips, baked potatoes, or low-fat muffins."

Yet fat does not raise your blood sugar. Carbohydrates do. The commonly recommended "diabetic diet" depends on medication, usually in increasing doses. Even then, it generally does not create normal blood sugar, and the "control" achieved still leads too often to crippling, even life-threatening, complications.

What is truly normal blood sugar? Diabetes Education Online, a resource from the University of California, San Francisco, tells us that "overnight and between meals, the normal, non-diabetic blood sugar ranges between 60 and 100 mg/dL [3.3 and 5.5 mmol/L] and 140 mg/dL [7.8 mmol/L] or less after meals and snacks."

Yet the target blood sugar ranges for people with diabetes listed by both the Joslin Diabetes Center and the American Diabetes Association go as high as 130 mg/dL (7.2 mmol/L) for fasting blood sugar, and up to 180 mg/dL (10 mmol/L) after meals or snacks. It is these levels that lead to widespread damage in people with "controlled" diabetes.

There is a depressing assumption in the medical community that people with diabetes will inevitably end up with at least some complications. This is because they do. The illnesses listed earlier are occurring in people with diabetes treated according to current guidelines. One frightening example: The National Institute of Diabetes and Digestive and Kidney Diseases states, "Even when diabetes is controlled, the disease can lead to CKD [chronic kidney disease] and kidney failure." That's a frightening definition of "controlled," because—and be clear on this—these debilitating, life-altering repercussions are expected in people with diabetes who are being treated according to the current standards.

Richard K. Bernstein, M.D., a physician with type 1 diabetes and a longtime advocate of carbohydrate restriction for glucose control, nailed it when he said, "The ADA (American Diabetes Association) has repeatedly advocated by their blood sugar and A1c guidelines that DIABETICS ARE NOT ENTITLED TO THE SAME BLOOD SUGARS AS NON-DIABETICS [Bernstein's emphasis] and thus should be destined to suffer the morbidity and mortality caused by high blood sugars. They ensure this sad outcome by advocating high carbohydrate diets and industrial doses of medication to cover the carbs and thereby cause both very high and very low (not normal) blood sugars."

HOW CAN I AVOID THIS FATE?

You must normalize your blood sugar. Not just control it, normalize it. Despite what you may have been told, this is not only possible, but simpler than most people—including most doctors—imagine.

If you have been diagnosed with diabetes or prediabetes, you are profoundly carbohydrate intolerant. This is what diabetes is: an inability to safely metabolize carbohydrates. It is bewildering to us that so many authorities recommend a low-fat diet rich in carbohydrates for people with diabetes, prescribing medication to "cover" the carbohydrate intake. We see this as akin to giving a peanut-allergic child a peanut butter sandwich and then injecting him with epinephrine and giving him steroids. It makes no sense. It is a losing game.

We at HEAL have a simpler, more elegant solution: Stop eating what's making you sick.

HEAL patients achieve actual, normal blood glucose levels—and with them, the cessation of that "inevitable" damage.

ABOUT HEAL

HEAL president Eric C. Westman, M.D., M.H.S., is America's top researcher in the study of the effects of carbohydrate restriction and a ketogenic diet (more on that later) on type 2 diabetes, having run Duke University's Lifestyle Medicine Clinic for nearly ten years after spending ten years doing clinical research. From his extensive experience comes one simple principle, which is the core of the HEAL Protocol: Axe the carbohydrates from the diet, and blood sugar normalizes, drastically reducing or even eliminating the chances of long-term complications.

HEAL Diabetes & Medical Weight Loss Clinics are the outgrowth of Dr. Westman's research and clinical experience, and his determination to bring his simple but profound low-carbohydrate protocol to people across the United States.

HEAL also draws on the vast experience of Jacqueline Eberstein, R.N. For thirty years, she was the director of medical education at the Atkins Center for Complementary Medicine. During that time, she supervised the treatment of thousands of people with diabetes by slashing their carbohydrate intake to 20 grams per day.

Dr. Westman first saw carbohydrate restriction used in a clinical setting when he visited the Atkins Center in 1999, after observing its success in a few of his patients. It changed the course of his career. He met Robert C. Atkins, M.D., and Jackie Eberstein and persuaded Dr. Atkins to fund clinical research on low-carbohydrate diets. That research led to the HEAL Protocol.

According to Dr. Westman, the link is a no-brainer: "It's taught in Physiology 101 that what raises blood sugar is carbohydrates in the diet. There's no controversy about that." Accordingly, Dr. Westman started putting people with diabetes on a very low-carbohydrate diet—with a daily maximum of just 20 grams of carbohydrate.

The result? To date, 95 percent of people with diabetes who stick to the protocol achieve *normal* blood sugar, 100 mg/dL (5.5 mmol/L) or less, while reducing or eliminating the need for medication; 75 percent eliminate medication entirely.

You don't have to wince at every step. You don't have to go blind. You don't have to wind up on dialysis, undergo a foot amputation, or die young. You don't. You can be well—free of the constant worry and the medical treadmill. You can have normal blood sugar.

All you have to do is stop eating what's making you sick.

THE HEAL PROTOCOL IN A NUTSHELL

At HEAL Diabetes & Medical Weight Loss Clinics, people with diabetes are prescribed a diet containing only 20 grams of carbohydrate per day. This means no starches and no sugars—those 20 grams come from just a couple of cups of salad or nonstarchy vegetables per day.

At the same time, HEAL medical advisors dramatically cut medication, because dosages of diabetes medications are based on the assumption that patients will be eating carbs. It is HEAL's aim to have people with diabetes completely medication free, with normal blood sugar. Not controlled blood sugar. Normal blood sugar.

AREN'T CARBS ESSENTIAL?

The short-form answer is no. But I'll elaborate.

In nutrition, "essential" has a specific meaning: Your body must have it *and* cannot make it itself no matter what other nutrients you eat. Your body needs a little bit of glucose (the simple sugar we mean when we say "blood sugar"), it's true, but only a very little bit; a healthy person should have only 5 grams of glucose in his or her bloodstream at any time. That's just over a teaspoon. Your body can easily make this much glucose in your liver, a process called gluconeogenesis. (Indeed, many people with diabetes are all too good at gluconeogenesis; this is what causes elevated blood sugar on rising, often called the "dawn effect.")

On the HEAL program, you will shift from being a sugar-burner to being a fat-burner, converting free fatty acids and ketones into energy. The medical term for this dietary approach is "ketogenic diet."

WHAT IS A KETOGENIC DIET?

A ketogenic diet is a diet that causes an increase in ketones, a.k.a. ketone bodies, in the bloodstream. So what are ketones? The Joslin Diabetes Center uses this definition: "Ketones are produced when the body burns fat for energy or fuel."

A ketogenic diet shifts the body to burning fat for fuel. We do this by removing carbohydrates, which are overwhelmingly the main source of glucose. You've read that various exercise programs will put you in your "fat-burning zone"? There's a more direct route: Stop giving your body carbohydrates, and it will adjust and start burning fat for fuel. Ketones are a breakdown product of that process and are also a form of fuel.

However, many people misguidedly believe that ketones are dangerous and even poisonous because they are usually discussed in the context of insulin-dependent diabetes, in the form of *ketoacidosis*. For example, the Joslin Diabetes Center states: "Without enough insulin, glucose builds up in the blood. Since the body is unable to use glucose for energy, it breaks down fat instead. When this occurs, ketones form in the blood and spill into the urine. These ketones can make you very sick." In this condition, not only are ketone levels elevated far beyond levels induced by carbohydrate restriction, but blood glucose levels are also dangerously elevated. In addition, the blood becomes acidic.

Nutritional or dietary ketosis is a distinct condition. Because carbohydrates are strictly limited, blood sugar cannot rise dangerously. There is no runaway buildup of ketones, sugar, or acids in the blood.

Because modern diets revolve around grains and sugars, there has been an assumption that glucose is the "normal" fuel of the body. But ketones are produced any time you burn fat for fuel, and any time you fast, even just overnight. If you are burning fat, you are producing ketones. The more of your fuel you derive from fat, the more ketones you will create. The Joslin Diabetes Center also advises, "Positive ketones are not a problem when blood glucose levels are within range and you are trying to lose weight." This is exactly the condition you want.

In the *Journal of the International Society of Sports Nutrition*, we find this useful description: "During very low carbohydrate intake, the regulated and controlled production of ketone bodies causes a harmless physiological state known as dietary ketosis. Ketone bodies flow from the liver to extra-hepatic tissues (e.g., brain) for use as a fuel; this spares glucose metabolism via a mechanism similar to the sparing of glucose by oxidation of fatty acids as an alternative fuel. In comparison with glucose, the ketone bodies are actually a very good respiratory fuel. *Indeed, there is no clear requirement for dietary carbohydrates for human adults.*" (My italics.)

One more thing about ketones, and a cheerful thing it is: They suppress appetite, often to a remarkable degree. Sure makes it easier to walk past the doughnuts.

WARNING: YOU NEED A DOCTOR'S SUPERVISION

If you have been diagnosed with diabetes, do not just jump in and start following the HEAL Protocol on your own. This diet is powerful medicine, and it will profoundly affect your metabolism—for the good—but it is still a major change.

If you are managing your diabetes with medication, your dosages have been prescribed based on the assumption that you will eat a certain quantity of carbohydrate foods with each meal. If you simply stop eating carbohydrates while continuing medication, you risk severe hypoglycemia (abnormally low blood sugar), even insulin shock. This is potentially fatal. For this reason, *it is imperative that you be under a doctor's supervision while making this transition.*

At HEAL Clinics, it is standard to both discontinue oral hypoglycemic drugs and halve insulin dosages from the first day. From there, blood sugar is closely monitored, and drugs adjusted up or down as needed. A doctor's supervision is essential during this process.

If you are not on medication, and do not yet have true diabetes, go ahead and cut out carbs. It's a wonderfully healthful way to eat. And no, you won't wind up "carb deficient."

WILL I LOSE WEIGHT?

Almost certainly. Repeated clinical trials have shown that very low-carbohydrate diets cause weight loss and—even better—get results at a higher calorie intake than necessary for weight loss with a low-fat diet.

In 1956, a pair of British researchers named Kekwick and Pawan published in *The Lancet* their groundbreaking study of the effect of the kind of calories eaten—carbohydrate, protein, or fat—on weight loss. They found that patients could gain a little weight on 1,000 calories per day of carbohydrate, while losing a bit on 1,000 calories per day of protein, and losing far more on 1,000 calories per day of fat. The same patients, when the diet was liberalized, would maintain or even gain weight on 2,000 calories per day of a "mixed" or "balanced" diet, but would lose weight easily on 2,600 calories per day of a protein and fat diet, with very little carbohydrate. For those of you who have struggled miserably to lose weight on 1,200 calories per day, this is very good news indeed.

In 1971, the *American Journal of Clinical Nutrition* published a study of moderately obese college men assigned to diets that had the same calorie count—1,800 per day—and the same amount of protein. However, one group got 104 grams of carbohydrate per day, another 60 grams, and the third 30 grams. The result? "Weight loss, fat loss, and percent weight lost as fat appeared to be inversely related to the level of carbohydrate in the isocaloric, isoprotein diets. No adequate explanation can be given for weight loss differences." In other words, with calorie and protein intakes kept identical, the lower the carbohydrate intake, the greater the weight and fat loss—and the researchers did not know why.

In a 2003 study of obese adolescents at Schneider's Children's Hospital in New York, kids were given either a low-fat diet or a low-carbohydrate diet for twelve weeks. The low-carb eaters lost twice as much weight as those in the low-fat group, while eating, on average, 60 percent more calories. Kids have an edge, since they're growing, but that's still a heck of a difference.

Despite the old refrain of "a calorie is a calorie is a calorie," we have ample evidence that the body, being a complex living system, reacts differently to different kinds of calories, and that carbohydrate restriction gives a metabolic edge.

Add to this three other things:

You'll be getting access to all that stored fuel you've been carrying around. As your insulin levels drop, your body will relearn how to use that fuel and will finally start to burn it.

If you have genuine, physical addictions to some carbohydrate foods, most commonly sugar and wheat, consuming the addictive substance only drives further cravings. Cut the addictive substance out, and physical sanity will reinstate itself.

And you will be less hungry. Between the satiating effects of protein and fat, the stabilization of your blood sugar so you no longer are battling crashes, and the appetite-killing effects of ketones, you are likely to find that you are automatically eating the right quantity of food for your body. Combine that with the metabolic advantage of a low-carbohydrate diet, and the weight will start coming off.

NOT JUST SUGAR

Because of the term "blood sugar," many believe that sugar is the enemy. It is, but not the only one. All carbohydrates are composed of sugar. Starches—potatoes, bread, cereal, and the like—are simply a lot of sugar molecules strung together. Digestion quickly converts them to glucose. Starches raise your blood sugar as much as any sugar. Doubt it? The journal *Diabetes Care* states that whole-wheat bread will raise your blood sugar more rapidly than an equivalent quantity of table sugar. Yikes.

This means that many foods you have considered healthful are not. The starches suggested

by the National Institutes of Health in their booklet *What I Need to Know about Eating and Diabetes* —including bread, potatoes, tortillas, pasta, rice, corn, crackers, yams, pretzels, and cereal—all will spike your blood sugar as much as, or more than, an equivalent quantity of table sugar.

How about fruit, juice, honey, and natural sugars? They're still sugars. No matter the source, a glucose molecule is a glucose molecule.

KEEP YOUR EYE ON THE BALL

There is so much nutritional advice coming at us —"Eat organic!, "Gluten-free is a fad!" "Don't eat anything with a list of ingredients!" "Only local, grass-fed meat and dairy!" Et cetera, ad confusionem.

For the moment, ignore it all. You have just one job: Keep your total carb intake to 20 grams per day or fewer. That's it.

I'm not saying that none of that endless advice has merit. I, by way of example, buy grass-fed butter, raise my eggs in my backyard, and don't eat gluten.

But I have been eating this way for twenty years now. I'm comfortable with it. I'm clear on what is and is not loaded with carbs. You, on the other hand, are a newbie. Focus on carbs. Just carbs.

Do not let yourself be fooled into thinking that apple juice is better than diet soda, because "it's natural!" Just 1 cup (240 ml) of apple juice contains 29 grams of sugar. Organic sugar from a natural source is still sugar and will still raise your blood glucose and worsen insulin resistance. Don't buy gluten-free bread, figuring that gluten-free also means low carbohydrate. It does not. Agave nectar is not better than sucralose (Splenda) because it's "natural" and "low glycemic" (meaning it raises blood sugar slowly). It is full of fructose (fruit sugar), which worsens insulin resistance.

Remember: 20 grams of total carbs per day. That is your metric, your focus, your goal. If you do this, your blood sugar will drop like pine needles the week after Christmas, we promise.

WHAT ABOUT NET CARBS?

You'll see a lot written about "net carbs." What does this mean?

As first proposed by Michael Eades, M.D., and Mary Dan Eades, M.D., in their book *Protein Power*, the idea was simple: Because fiber is a carbohydrate, but one that the human gut can neither digest nor absorb, dieters could subtract the grams of fiber in a food from the total carb count to get the number of grams of carbohydrate that actually wind up in the bloodstream. This was a way to let their patients eat more vegetables, and maybe a few berries or a little melon.

But you know how it is: Give people an exception to the rule, and they start working out ways to game the system. Pretty soon food processors were subtracting all sorts of things from the total carb count: maltitol, low-glycemic-index sugars, glycerin, resistant starch, you name it. This led to an explosion of foods with "net carb" counts that can best be described as dubious. Many people embraced these products only to find they were not losing weight or getting any of the other benefits of a low-carbohydrate diet.

Also to be considered is that even if, as the Eades intended, you get your carbohydrates from vegetables and low-sugar fruit, you still get more digestible, absorbable carbohydrate than when counting total carbs. Since the Eades were concerned with weight loss, this was not of great concern.

But we are talking about diabetes, end-stage carbohydrate intolerance. We are not talking about looking better at the high school reunion (although you will). We're talking about reversing very serious illness. We're talking about avoiding painful nerve damage, amputated limbs, blindness, heart disease, kidney failure, and early death. We're talking about your life.

It is common for diet plans to make allowances for "cheating." And the ads on television give testament to all the ways people try to fool themselves into thinking that there is some "healthy" way to continue their addiction, from sugar-loaded "fiber bars" to sugar-loaded "fruit" punch with a few added vitamins. You cannot afford this. Every time your blood sugar goes above 120 mg/dL (6.7 mmol/L) your body sustains irreversible damage, and that damage adds up. Every time you fall for this nonsense, you will move a little closer to disastrous consequences.

This is scary stuff. We have no wiggle room. This is why, at HEAL, we count total carbs, not net carbs. There may come a day when you can afford to loosen up a tiny bit and count net carbs, but until and unless your doctor gives you the green light, that day has not arrived.

Ignore net carb counts. Count total carbs.

However, for those of you who do not have diabetes and are simply restricting carbs for weight loss and health, we've included fiber counts along with total carb counts. Simple subtraction will give you the net carb counts.

ISN'T SUCH AN UNBALANCED DIET SHORT ON VITAMINS AND MINERALS?

In a word, no, though we certainly suggest you eat a wide variety of the allowed foods.

Animal products and vegetables are among the most nutrient-dense foods. There is no vitamin or mineral in starchy foods that cannot be found in low-carbohydrate foods.

Brown rice, long a darling of the health food set, is a great example. One-half cup of cooked brown rice has 109 calories, with 23 grams of carbohydrate. How nutritious is it? It will contain:

0% of the daily value of vitamin A

6% of the daily value of vitamin B_1 (thiamine)

1% of the daily value of vitamin B_2 (riboflavin)

6% of the daily value of vitamin B_3 (niacin)

7% of the daily value of vitamin B_6 (pyridoxine)

0% of the daily value of vitamin B_{12}

1% of the daily value of folacin

0% of the daily value of vitamin C

1% of the daily value of calcium

3% of the daily value of iron (in a poorly absorbed form)

1% of the daily value of potassium

4% of the daily value of zinc

One cup of **romaine lettuce** has a mere 8 calories, with 1 gram of carbohydrate. Yet it contains:

29% of the daily value of vitamin A

4% of the daily value of vitamin B_1

3% of the daily value of vitamin B_2

1% of the daily value of vitamin B_3

1% of the daily value of vitamin B_6

0% of the daily value of vitamin B_{12}

19% of the daily value of folacin

22% of the daily value of vitamin C

2% of the daily value of calcium

3% of the daily value of iron

5% of the daily value of potassium

1% of the daily value of zinc

How about **whole-wheat pasta**? Three-quarters of a cup (66 g) of dry whole-wheat pasta—about 1¼ cups (210 g) cooked—will have 274 calories and 59 grams of carbohydrate. It will provide:

0% of the daily value of vitamin A

26% of the daily value of vitamin B_1

7% of the daily value of vitamin B_2

20% of the daily value of vitamin B_3

9% of the daily value of vitamin B_6

0% of the daily value of vitamin B_{12}

11% of the daily value of folacin

0% of the daily value of vitamin C

3% of the daily value of calcium

16% of the daily value of iron

5% of the daily value of potassium

12% of the daily value of zinc

Compare this with a 6-ounce (170 g) **salmon fillet** sautéed in a little butter. It will have 299 calories and a mere trace of carbohydrate. With it you will get:

17% of the daily value of vitamin A

23% of the daily value of vitamin B_1

13% of the daily value of vitamin B_2

43% of the daily value of vitamin B_3

17% of the daily value of vitamin B_6

85% of the daily value of vitamin B_{12}

2% of the daily value of folacin

3% of the daily value of calcium
7% of the daily value of iron
16% of the daily value of potassium
6% of the daily value of zinc

Need a snack? You could have an **apple**, for 81 calories and 21 grams of carbohydrate. It will provide:

1% of the daily value of vitamin A
1% of the daily value of vitamin B_1
1% of the daily value of vitamin B_2
1% of the daily value of vitamin B_3
3% of the daily value of vitamin B_6
0% of the daily value of vitamin B_{12}
1% of the daily value of folacin
1% of the daily value of calcium
1% of the daily value of iron
5% of the daily value of potassium
0% of the daily value of zinc

Or you could have an "**unsandwich**" of a slice each of ham and cheese, with a little mustard or mayo or both in between. Exclusive of condiments, you'll get 166 calories and 1 gram of carbohydrate, along with:

9% of the daily value of vitamin A
17% of the daily value of vitamin B_1
10% of the daily value of vitamin B_2
8% of the daily value of vitamin B_3
6% of the daily value of vitamin B_6
8% of the daily value of vitamin B_{12}
2% of the daily value of folacin
21% of the daily value of calcium
3% of the daily value of iron
3% of the daily value of potassium
10% of the daily value of zinc

(I'm going to insert this, because it's such a persistent myth: You don't need to eat bananas—28 grams of carbohydrate apiece—to get potassium. One banana has 13 percent of your potassium for the day. A 6-ounce [170 g] pork chop will provide 14 percent; 6 ounces [170 g] of sole fillet will provide 18 percent; 6 [170 g] ounces of beef chuck provides 13 percent; half an avocado provides 17 percent. I can only assume that bananas have a good press agent.)

This isn't even considering outright junk—chips, candy, etc. You know that stuff doesn't add to your daily nutrition. In fact, it can dilute it by displacing nutritious foods.

There is no essential vitamin or mineral yet identified that is not available from low-carbohydrate sources—and many grain foods only appear to have a good nutritional profile because they've been enriched at the factory. Enrichment was instituted when it became clear that people whose diets depended on milled grains were developing nutritional deficiency diseases.

It is likely that your nutritional profile will improve. That said, we do recommend taking a well-formulated, iron-free multivitamin daily.

WHAT ABOUT "GOOD CARBS"?

No doubt you've heard that there are "good carbs." It may come as a shock, then, to learn that once they are digested and absorbed there is chemically no difference between one source of sugar and another. A molecule of glucose derived from brown rice is identical to a molecule of glucose derived from a convenience store slushy. The brown rice brings a few vitamins along with it, but the glucose is the same. It all will do the same thing to your blood sugar. It all will cause the same damage.

Nonstarchy vegetables are "good carbs" largely because they actually contain very little carbohydrate along with their substantial amounts of vitamins, minerals, and antioxidants.

AREN'T CARBS ENERGY FOOD?

This is the very opposite of the truth, so wrong-headed as to be funny if it weren't making so many lives miserable. Americans are practically bathing in carbs, yet fatigue is one of the most common medical complaints.

Perhaps you have heard that carbs are "quick energy." This is exactly what is wrong with them. Consider an analogy: Gasoline is quick energy, so quick that if you were to check your gas tank by match light, you'd be lucky to live to tell about it. That's why your car has fuel injectors or a carburetor—to give it a way to use that explosively quick energy gradually. Without it? *Ka-boom.*

Your body doesn't have a carburetor. It has no way to use carbohydrates gradually. When you eat a carb-heavy meal, it is rapidly converted into glucose and rushes into your bloodstream. Your blood sugar shoots up. Your body knows that this is dangerous, so it cranks out lots of insulin to bring your blood sugar down. It converts that sugar to fats known as triglycerides, and stuffs them into your fat cells.

A few things happen: You have some new fat around your waist, and possibly in your liver. Your triglycerides have gone up. And your blood sugar has crashed as quickly as it rose, leaving you tired, cranky, and *hungry.*

Your body should be able to use that new fat for fuel. Storage fat should be your steady fuel supply, so that when you burn through the calories in your last meal, you shift over to burning stored fuel with no drop in energy or efficiency. But falling insulin levels are the body's signal to let that stored fat out into the bloodstream, and those carbs you are eating ensure that your insulin is going nowhere but up.

So you eat carbs, and your blood sugar rises sharply. Your body sends out insulin to get your blood sugar back down, shunting most of the fuel you just ate into storage as fat and locking it up. Your blood sugar falls, and you get tired, foggy-headed, irritable, and hungry. You grab a muffin, and the whole process starts over.

As this cycle is endlessly repeated, the insulin receptors—the little "doors" on your cells that the insulin "opens" to usher the sugar out of your bloodstream—start to wear out. You make more and more insulin, and yet it gets harder and harder for your body to get your blood sugar down. Cue the diagnosis of diabetes.

Here's the irony of "energy food": You're carrying around all the fuel you need to get you through weeks, possibly months, but because of high insulin levels you can't get to it. Yet you still have to lug it around everywhere you go. No wonder you're tired and hungry all the time.

Fat is the real energy food. That 1 teaspoon of sugar in a healthy bloodstream should be the tinder. Fat is the big darned logs that burn for hours and hours. And since you carry a supply of fat around with you, once your insulin levels drop and you get access to the "tank," you'll have steady, near inexhaustible energy. When you burn through the fat in your last meal, you'll shift smoothly over to burning body fat with no mid-morning slump. That's how the system is supposed to work. With access to all that stored fuel, and no more blood sugar roller coaster, you'll find that you are less hungry. You may be shocked at how much your appetite is reduced.

All you have to do is stop the cycle. Breaking it won't make you tired and hungry. Instead, you will have more energy and less hunger that you ever imagined possible.

This is how your body evolved to work: Store fuel when it's plentiful and then tap into those reserves in between times. How else do you think your hunter-gatherer ancestors tracked a mammoth when they hadn't eaten in a couple of days? It's an elegant system.

KETO FLU

You may, however, have a few days of "keto flu." What is keto flu? It's analogous to drug withdrawal. Here's the deal.

Your body knows that high blood sugar is dangerous. If your blood sugar is elevated, so is your insulin, because your body is trying like heck to get rid of that sugar. This means that your body will always burn glucose before it gets around to burning fat for fuel. (This is how so many people got the mistaken idea that glucose is the primary fuel of the body.)

If you've been giving your body carbohydrate every few hours—cereal for breakfast, a doughnut on break, fries with your lunch, etc.—your body rarely gets around to burning fat. According to an article in the *Journal of Lipid Research*, insulin signals your body to reduce production of the enzyme needed to release fat from cells to be burned. Since you rarely use it, you make less of the stuff.

So when you stop eating carbs, your body may be confused for a few days—you're not giving it glucose, and it's having trouble releasing fat. You may be tired, achy, or have trouble concentrating. Do not panic. Do not give up. If you quit a two-pack-a-day cigarette habit and felt bad for a few days,

would you assume it meant that giving up smoking was a bad idea? Same thing here. Your body *will* step up production of the enzymes needed to burn fat for fuel.

SODIUM

Another reason people can feel a little off in the first week or two is dehydration from salt and water loss. Salt has been so demonized that you may be unaware that it is—unlike carbohydrate—an essential nutrient.

The *American Journal of Physiology* tells us that high insulin levels signal the kidneys to hang on to sodium, and with it water, even to the point of causing high blood pressure. When you go low carb and your insulin levels drop, your kidneys get the signal to let that sodium go, along with the water it holds. This is why most people drop several pounds of water weight in the first few days, and high blood pressure comes down quickly.

Because of this, it is possible to wind up with dehydration and low sodium levels, especially as you'll also be cutting out most high-sodium processed food. The symptoms of dehydration include light-headedness, fatigue, headaches, muscle aches, and possibly cramps.

It's easy to prevent this. Don't hesitate to use salt in cooking and at the table, and if you feel weak, dizzy, or achy, add a cup or two of bouillon or heavily salted broth per day. The salt and water in the bouillon will replace some of the salt and water that you have lost, and you'll feel better in just 10 minutes.

DO I NEED TO EXERCISE?

If you want to exercise, great. But we're not going to push you. Until you shift over to a fat- and ketone-burning metabolism and get access to the tank, you're likely to be tired. You should feel your energy level rise as your body adjusts. If you find yourself wanting to go for a walk, go dancing, take a yoga class, or lift weights—we're all for it. But don't make yourself miserable.

And remember: You cannot exercise your way out of a lousy diet.

WON'T A HIGH-FAT DIET GIVE ME HEART DISEASE?

First, know this: Diabetes will give you heart disease. Remember, people with diabetes have double the risk of heart disease compared with those who do not have the condition. That includes all those people who are "controlling" their diabetes according to current standards.

BUT WHAT ABOUT CHOLESTEROL? TRIGLYCERIDES?

The issue of triglycerides is clear-cut: High levels of triglycerides, widely accepted as an important marker of heart disease, are driven not by fat intake, but by carbohydrate intake. In *Current Opinion in Lipidology*, we find this clear statement: "High-carbohydrate/low-fat, isocaloric [neither high nor low calorie] diets have repeatedly been shown to increase plasma triglyceride concentrations. Indeed, there is a medical term for this: carbohydrate-induced hypertriglyceridemia."

Knowing this, it is no surprise that triglyceride levels drop, often precipitously, on a low-carbohydrate diet.

HOW ABOUT CHOLESTEROL?

We trust that by now you've gathered that the cholesterol issue is more complicated than your total cholesterol number. You've likely heard of LDL cholesterol, often called "bad" cholesterol, and HDL, considered "good" cholesterol. Most doctors look at the ratios of these to one another, to total cholesterol, and to triglycerides. What does a low-carbohydrate, high-fat diet do to these ratios?

A 2014 study at Tulane University in New Orleans compared a low-carbohydrate diet with a low-fat diet in a yearlong trial. The low-carb dieters were to eat 40 grams or fewer of carbohydrate per day, while the low-fat dieters were told to get 30 percent or less of their calories from fat. What happened?

The low-carbohydrate group had greater improvements in HDL cholesterol and triglyceride levels, and in the ratio of total cholesterol to HDL. Their estimated ten-year heart disease risk declined.

But these were nonobese, nondiabetic subjects. What about people who are already ill?

A 2007 study of a ketogenic diet—very low carbohydrate and high fat—looked at the effects on both obese yet healthy subjects and obese subjects with high blood sugar. After fifty-six weeks, the study showed that total cholesterol, LDL, and triglycerides all showed a "significant decrease," while HDL increased significantly. The researchers noted that these changes were actually more significant in subjects who started with high blood glucose.

The kicker? There were also reductions in blood sugar, along with body weight and body mass index.

But the implications are far wider. Low-carb, high-fat ketogenic diets, first used medically for diabetes control in 1797 by John Rollo, a Scottish military surgeon, and for seizure control in the early twentieth century, are showing promise for treating many health problems.

- A study published in 2011 in the scientific journal *PLOS One* looked at the effects of a ketogenic diet on diabetic nephropathy—the most common cause of kidney failure—in diabetic mice. The result? Two months on a ketogenic diet actually reversed kidney damage. This has hitherto been virtually unheard of.

- In August 2013, the *Clinical Journal of the American Society of Nephrology* published the results of a small human trial, again showing an improvement in kidney function in people with type 2 diabetes with nephropathy after twelve weeks on a ketogenic diet.

- In 2012, in the journal *Nutrition*, Richard D. Feinman, M.D., and Eugene Fine, M.D., published groundbreaking work regarding the effectiveness of such diets in inhibiting cancer growth by reducing insulin signaling.

- A 2014 article in *BioMed Research International* states: "[The] ketogenic diet is recognized as an effective treatment for pharmacoresistant epilepsy but emerging data suggests that ketogenic diets could be also useful in amyotrophic lateral sclerosis, Alzheimer, Parkinson's disease, and some mitochondriopathies [disorders of the mitochondria, the energy-producing powerhouses of the cells]."

- A 2014 article in the *Journal of Child Neurology* looked at the power of ketogenic diets to reduce pain, finding a long-term reduction in pain in rats. The article states that "many types of pain and painful or progressive conditions involve chronic inflammation" and "several mechanistic threads support the hypothesis that a ketogenic diet will reduce inflammation." Because inflammation is implicated in many illnesses, from heart disease to cancer, this is exciting news.

- In 2005, *Nutrition & Metabolism* published an article regarding a pilot study of a ketogenic diet for treatment of polycystic ovarian syndrome (PCOS), the leading cause of female infertility. The study found that the diet not only caused "significant" weight loss but also improved hormone balance and lowered fasting insulin.

- In a 2010 interview for the Cureality blog, Michael Fox, M.D., a reproductive endocrinologist specializing in fertility problems, states, "We now recommend the VLCD [very low-carbohydrate diet] to all fertility patients and their spouses. The pregnancy rates do seem much better overall, as well as seeing a reduction in miscarriage rates."

CHAPTER 2
So What Can I Eat?

It's all well and good to tell you to eat 20 grams or fewer of carbohydrate per day. But what does that mean? What can you eat?

First, divide up those carbs: You're shooting for 5 grams per meal, plus 5 grams in a snack. Do not eat all 20 grams at one meal. Five grams will barely budge your blood sugar. Twenty all together will probably raise it.

Eat at least three meals per day. Feeling full helps you resist the junk food that crosses your path and prevents you from stressing your body, which can cause an adrenaline release that can raise your blood sugar.

The heart of your diet will be meat, fish, poultry, eggs, cheese, nonstarchy vegetables, and natural fats—those that come along with your protein foods, such as the fat on steaks or the skin on chicken, plus butter, olive oil, coconut oil, peanut oil, lard, tallow, chicken fat, and the like. Let's dolly in for a close-up.

WHEN YOU ARE HUNGRY, YOU MAY EAT AS MUCH AS YOU WANT OF THESE

- Any unprocessed meat: Beef (ground beef, steak, etc.), pork, lamb, veal, or other meats. If you have a hunter in the family, feel free to eat any kind of game.

- These processed meats: Breakfast sausage, bacon, pepperoni, hot dogs, many cold cuts, and ham. These generally have a small quantity of sugar added. Read the labels and choose those with the lowest sugar content. There are hot dogs with 1 gram of carbohydrate and hot dogs with 4 grams of carbohydrate (same thing with ham). Choose the lowest carb brands you can find.

- Poultry: Chicken, turkey, duck, Cornish game hen, or any other fowl. Again, if you have a hunter in the family, feel free to eat any game bird.

- Fish and shellfish: Any fish, including tuna, salmon, catfish, cod, flounder, sole, red snapper, mahimahi, bass, and trout, as well as shrimp, scallops, crab, and lobster. Clams, oysters, and mussels have some naturally occurring carbohydrate in them, so choose them only occasionally.

- Eggs: Whole eggs are permitted without restriction. Eat the yolks!

ADD THESE FOODS

Vegetables

You will add to these core foods a couple of moderate portions of salad greens and/or nonstarchy vegetables per day.

Your choice of greens includes, but is not limited to: Arugula, bok choy, cabbage (all varieties), chard, chives, endive, greens (all varieties including beet, collards, mustard, and turnip), kale, lettuce (all varieties), parsley, spinach, radicchio, radishes, scallions, and watercress. If it is a leaf, you can eat it.

Nonstarchy vegetables include: Artichokes, asparagus, broccoli, Brussels sprouts, cauliflower, celery, cucumber, eggplant, green beans (string beans), jicama, leeks, mushrooms, okra, onions, peppers, pumpkin, shallots, snow peas, sprouts (bean and alfalfa), sugar-snap peas, summer squash, tomatoes, rhubarb, wax beans, zucchini.

Quantities of vegetables will vary a bit, since they contain differing quantities of carbohydrate. The recipes in this book take this into account. If you're simply making a salad, figure on 1 cup of loosely packed leaves; if you're having sautéed, roasted, or steamed vegetables, figure ½ to 1 cup of nonstarchy vegetables.

Fats—Yes, Fats

All fats and oils, even butter, are allowed. Olive oil and peanut oil are especially healthy oils and are encouraged in cooking. Natural fats that come with your food are allowed, along with coconut oil and lard (avoid hydrogenated lard).

Avoid margarine and other hydrogenated oils. It is best to minimize soy, corn, canola, and safflower oils. For salad dressings, use oil and vinegar, blue cheese, ranch, Caesar, or Italian. Avoid "lite" dressings, as these commonly have more carbohydrate. Chopped eggs, bacon, and grated cheese may also be included in salads.

Fats, in general, are important because they add flavor and make you feel full. Do not attempt to follow a low-fat diet!

It's common for people to refer to low-carbohydrate diets as "high protein," but you are actually shooting for a low-carbohydrate/moderate-protein /high-fat diet. Fat should be what makes up the calories you've subtracted by cutting carbohydrates. Understand that natural fats are not just "not bad," they're healthful. Eat the fat on your steaks and chops, egg yolks, and poultry skin. Feel free to eat delicious, fatty meats such as rib-eye steaks, spareribs, bacon, and duck. Fry or scramble your eggs in butter or bacon grease, sauté or roast your vegetables with plenty of fat, and be generous with olive oil on your salads.

If you choose one of the lower fat recipes in this book—one calling for, say, boneless, skinless chicken breast or a lean white fish—pair it with a higher-fat side dish.

ADD THESE, TOO

In addition to animal proteins, vegetables, and fats, you may have:

- Avocado: Up to one-half Hass avocado (the little pebbly-skinned black ones) per day. This is the one exception to the only-5-grams-at-a-time rule. Half a Hass avocado will have about 7 grams of carbohydrate, but they are so healthful—loaded with good fats, fiber, and potassium—and so satisfying, that we encourage you to eat them.

- Cheese: Up to 4 ounces (115 g) per day of cheeses such as Swiss, Cheddar, Brie, Camembert, blue cheese, mozzarella, and Gruyère. Also cream cheese and goat cheeses. Check the carbohydrate counts.
- Cream: Up to 3 tablespoons (45 ml) per day of heavy cream or sour cream.
- Mayonnaise
- Olives: Black or green, up to 10 per day.
- Pickles: Dill or sugar-free, up to 2 per day.
- Soy sauce: Up to 2 tablespoons (28 ml) a day.

After the second week you may add up to 1 ounce (28 g) per day of walnuts, pecans, Brazil nuts, pine nuts, or macadamias.

Allowable seasonings include:

- All individual spices and herbs
- Spice blends that contain no sugar; a dismaying number of them do, so read the labels.
- Horseradish: Read the labels and choose one with no sugar.
- Lemon and lime juice
- Mustard: Dijon, spicy brown, or yellow mustard. (No honey mustard, and check the labels on other mustards.)

Do not use ketchup (although eating 1 or 2 tablespoons (15 to 28 g) of Heinz Reduced Sugar Ketchup per day is allowed), steak sauce, barbecue sauce, or cocktail sauce.

Food may be baked, boiled, stir-fried, sautéed, roasted, fried (with no flour, breading, or cornmeal), grilled, or microwaved.

As mentioned, some people become dehydrated in the first few weeks of eating low carb and need extra sodium. Unless directed otherwise by your physician, you can have bouillon or broth with extra salt stirred in up to twice a day as needed during the first few weeks of the diet to minimize headache or fatigue. If you're tired, achy, or dizzy, this is the first thing to try.

DO NOT EAT

On this diet, no sugars (simple carbohydrates) and no starches (complex carbohydrates) are eaten. The only carbohydrates we encourage are the nutritionally dense, fiber-rich vegetables previously listed. Sugars are simple carbohydrates. Avoid: White sugar, brown sugar, honey, maple syrup, agave nectar, molasses, corn syrup, beer (contains barley malt), milk (contains lactose), yogurt, dairy substitutes, fruit juice, fruit, canned soups, ketchup, and other sweet condiments and relishes.

Starches are complex carbohydrates that break down into sugars. Avoid: Grains (even whole grains), rice, cereals, flour and flour-containing items, cornstarch, breads, pastas, muffins, bagels, crackers, starchy vegetables such as legumes (pinto, lima, black beans, etc.), carrots, parsnips, corn, peas, potatoes, french fries, and potato chips etc.

BE WARY OF

Beware of fat-free or "lite" diet products; all too often the fat has been replaced with sugars, starches, or both. Anyway, you're not limiting your fat intake, remember? Also avoid sugar-free cookies and cakes—"sugar-free" does not mean "carb-free." Be careful of prepared dishes such as coleslaw; they often have sugar. At the deli or restaurant, ask questions, and remember, if it tastes sweet, and you don't know for certain it's from carb-free sweeteners, it's sugary.

Check the labels of liquid medications, cough syrups, cough drops, and other over-the-counter medications that may contain sugar. Most pharmacies carry "diabetic cough syrup" and cold-and-flu relief products in capsule, rather than liquid, form.

Avoid products that are labeled "Great for Low-Carb Diets!" and ignore "net carb counts." It's astonishing the garbage food processors try to rationalize.

Become an obsessive label reader. It is often bewildering the places sugar sneaks in. I once made the mistake of buying canned clams without reading the label, only to notice later they had added sugar. Who put sugar in the clams?

IT IS NOT ABOUT HOW MUCH YOU EAT

The HEAL Protocol is not about *how much* you eat; it is about *what* you eat. If you are hungry, eat! Have a hard-boiled egg, a chunk of cheese, a few chicken wings, a bunless cheeseburger. Eat when you are hungry. Stop when you are satisfied. Repeat.

However, if a food is not on the HEAL Protocol, it is out. Completely out.

On low-calorie diets, people are always making deals—"I'll skip 300 calories at lunch so I can have cake at the party later." This kind of deal does not work. No matter what healthy food you skip, that cake is going to jack your blood sugar through the roof. You'll be knocked out of ketosis—hunger renewed, back to addiction and craving—and it will take you the better part of a week to get back in the happy biochemical state where your hunger and cravings are suppressed and your blood sugar is rock-steady.

Just accept it: There is no way to play games with this nutritional protocol. There is no cheating. The word "cheat" implies that you'll get away with something, and you never will. Your body will know.

However, if you do deviate from your plan, get right back on the wagon with the next meal or snack. Do not decide, "I blew it at lunch, I may as well go ahead and have ice cream." Remember, every excess glucose molecule does damage. Ask yourself: If you stumbled on the top step, would you throw yourself down the stairs?

WHAT ABOUT "MODERATION"?

There will be people who try to derail you, intoning, "I believe in moderation in all things." They'll go on to say, "You should be able to have a treat now and then." They sound oh-so-reasonable.

Ask yourself: If you quit a two-pack-a-day cigarette habit, would you expect to be able to have just a couple on the weekend? If an alcoholic friend sobered up, would you tell him he was too rigid, and he should be able to have a glass or two of wine at a holiday dinner?

You're overcoming a serious, dangerous health issue, as deadly as smoking or alcoholism. Ignore those who would make light of it. It's not their feet, eyes, or kidneys at risk.

MENU PLANNING

The part of low-carb menu planning that takes getting used to is that it is difficult to have more than two dishes—a protein and a vegetable—within the constraints of 5 grams of carbohydrate per meal. Yet there is no need to go hungry. Remember, you may eat the listed animal foods to your heart's content, and add fat liberally—oil on your salad, butter on your vegetables or on your steak or seafood.

The most basic HEAL meal is an animal protein food—meat, poultry, fish, or eggs—cooked without added carbohydrate and paired with a nonstarchy vegetable. For instance:

- Broiled steak with sautéed mushrooms
- Roast chicken with asparagus and lemon butter
- Grilled salmon fillet with a green salad

But there are recipes in this book for meat, poultry, fish, or eggs combined with vegetables or seasonings that add as much as 5 grams of carbohydrate. Those you will have to eat solo. There are also recipes that have fewer than 5 grams. We are confident that you can add, and combine—or not combine—these dishes to wind up with 5 grams per meal.

WHAT ABOUT THE "CARBIVORES"?

You may well be cooking for "carbivores." What to do?

It's pretty simple. With the personal motto "I feed people, therefore I am," I have devised many menus that have allowed me to stick to my plan while making guests happy. The trick is to serve the starch separately. Look at those menus above. You can add baked potatoes to the steak with sautéed mushrooms, brown rice to the roast chicken with asparagus and lemon butter, or a few ears of grilled sweet corn along with the salmon. One word of advice: Don't choose your favorites. If you find rice boring but french fries irresistible, serve rice.

Look out for mixed dishes. If the family wants pasta, don't serve lasagna. Instead, make bread crumb–free meatballs, spaghetti, and no-sugar-added sauce, plus a salad with Italian vinaigrette. The family has spaghetti and meatballs and you have meatballs and a bit of sauce, with plenty of Parmesan cheese and salad on the side.

Do share your favorite low-carb dishes with your loved ones. Remember that your children share your DNA, and with it your risk of developing diabetes. The more you can encourage them to enjoy a healthy sugar-and-starch-free diet, the healthier they will be later in life. Some of the happiest emails I get are from parents telling me their children love my recipes.

WHAT ARE THE "NEXT STEP" RECIPES?

At the end of some chapters we have included Next Step recipes. These recipes have no more than 5 grams of carbohydrate per serving. So why the separate section?

Next Step recipes include ingredients that are not allowed in the early intervention stage of your recovery from diabetes. Usually they are ingredients that include some sugar—Worcestershire sauce, for instance—or fruit products, such as no-sugar-added preserves. These ingredients are used judiciously, of course, keeping within our 5-gram carb limit.

You need to wait until your doctor is confident your diabetes has been reversed to use the Next Step recipes, not because they'll spike your blood sugar—they won't—but because reintroducing these ingredients must be done cautiously. You need to learn to use them in limited quantities, for flavor, rather than adding them back willy-nilly.

Hooray! You have something more to look forward to!

 This logo identifies "NEXT STEP" recipes throughout the book.

WHAT'S FOR BREAKFAST?

The most common menu question we get is, "What can I have for breakfast?" Americans are used to grabbing something quick and carb heavy for breakfast—cereal, muffins, toast, etc.—and shifting gears seems a mammoth task. It doesn't have to be.

We urge you to eat breakfast. It keeps your blood sugar stable, but it's more important than that. If you'll be facing doughnuts in the break room, cake every time a colleague has a birthday, the smell of pizza wafting from the next cubicle, you need to be armed. Breakfast is your single most powerful weapon. Here are some ideas:

- Newsflash: You are not required to eat "breakfast food" for breakfast. You can eat anything you like —steak, a chop, tuna salad, chicken wings, you name it.

- Bacon, sausage, and ham are all fine, with or without eggs. Cook bacon or sausage in advance, and just give it a quick warm-up.

- An electric contact grill—you know, the George Foreman kind of thing—is hugely useful for cooking breakfast. You can throw in your bacon or sausage patties or a burger, and the meat will cook while you get dressed.

- Leftovers. I eat leftovers for breakfast often, anything from salad to meatloaf. The summer I wrote my barbecue book, I ate leftover chicken or ribs for breakfast every day for a couple of months.

- Eggs. If you like eggs, feel free to eat them daily, yolks and all—fried, scrambled, poached, in an omelet, whatever. The Insta-Quiche (page 63) or Confetti Frittata (page 62) both warm up nicely in the microwave. Hard-boiled eggs make a great grab-and-go breakfast.

- Make pancakes (page 53) or waffles (page 52) over the weekend, and freeze. Voilà! Toaster breakfast!

- Cheesecake makes a great breakfast, and this book has several. How decadent to have cheesecake for breakfast!

- Prewrapped cheese chunks are convenient for stashing in your purse or briefcase to eat on the go or at your desk.

- Can't face anything but coffee in the morning? See Power Pack Mocha and Morning Mocha, both on page 164.

FOR THOSE OF YOU WHO DON'T COOK

Yes, this is mainly a cookbook. Writing about convenience foods goes against the grain—pardon the pun—for me. I'm always nagging people to just cook something, will you, for crying out loud?! A little simple, plain cooking is your best defense against bad food, not to mention a sky-high food budget.

However, I am aware that many people rarely eat anything that takes more preparation than 3 minutes in the microwave or a trip through the drive-through. Even folks who do cook have days when they want something fast.

Most convenience food is as nutritionally bad as it is quick and easy. (Ironically, the Atkins brand frozen meals are too high carb for HEAL. Somewhere Dr. A is shaking his head sadly.) Still, there is real, decent food out there that takes almost no work, and it's not all bunless fast-food burgers.

- Rotisserie chicken: My local stores carry traditional, lemon-garlic, and barbecue. The barbecue flavor is most likely to have sugar. Leftover rotisserie chicken is great for chicken salad.

- Hot wings: Most have breading and sugar, but there are a few that squeak by. Pizza Hut Baked Hot Wings and Baked Mild Wings are both quite low carb. Choose the Buffalo sauce rather than the sugary barbecue sauce. Skip "boneless wings"—they're invariably breaded.

- Precooked bacon: If you hate preparing bacon, this is worth your money. Bacon without guilt is one of the great joys of low-carb eating.

- Frozen grilled fish fillets: Available in lemon pepper, garlic butter, Cajun, and more. Just microwave and eat.

- Frozen hamburger patties: Look for frozen burgers labeled "100% beef" to avoid fillers containing carbs and soy. Vary these by adding different kinds of cheese, sautéed mushrooms, bacon, a couple of teaspoons of minced onion, sprinkle-on seasonings, or what have you.

- Frozen cooked shrimp: Add these to a salad, or mix Heinz Reduced Sugar Ketchup with horseradish, lemon juice, and a shot of Tabasco to make cocktail sauce for dipping.

- Grilled chicken breast strips: Great in salads and omelets.

- Canned tuna, shrimp, crab, etc.: These are handy for dumping over a pile of greens for a quick main-dish salad. My husband will happily make a lunch of a simple can of sardines.

- Smoked salmon: Put this in a salad or an omelet, and you've gone beyond convenience food to elegance.

- Eggs: It's hard to spend more than 5 minutes frying or scrambling eggs. Hard-boil a dozen eggs over the weekend, stash 'em in the fridge, and they'll be there when you need a quick protein fix.

- Cold cuts: Identifiable cuts of meat, such as turkey breast, roast beef, and roasted or boiled ham are likely to have less sugar than things that are ground up and pressed back together, like bologna, chopped ham, and anything with "loaf" in the name. Read labels and ask questions. Try making those unsandwiches I mentioned earlier: Just spread mustard and mayo between a slice of meat and a slice of cheese, add a lettuce leaf if you like, roll it up, and eat.

- Individually wrapped cheese chunks: Swiss Knight, BabyBel, Laughing Cow, andstring cheese all make great grab-and-go snacks, or even breakfasts as previously mentioned. They're also great for stashing in a purse or carry-on bag while traveling.

- Deli salads and vegetables: These require some scouting. Skip the potato and macaroni salads. Sadly, coleslaw almost always contains sugar. But many grocery store delis carry at least a few things that work for us—tuna salad, chicken salad, even things like roasted asparagus. Do reconnaissance when you have a free 15 minutes, and the deli isn't slammed, so you can ask questions. In these food-allergy-conscious times, more and more delis post ingredient lists; read them.

- Ready-to-cook meat and fish: Many grocery stores carry kabobs and seasoned pork chops or fish, already prepped to take home and run under the broiler. Be wary about ingredients, and ask questions. If possible, do your shopping at a grocery store with a real meat department, not just prewrapped cuts.

- Thin cuts of meat: If you're short on time, buy thin pork chops and steaks. Unsurprisingly, they cook faster than thick ones.

- Bagged salad: Great stuff! Try a new blend from time to time. Also useful are coleslaw mix—

basically shredded cabbage—and prewashed baby spinach. Use it in salads but also try sautéing it lightly in olive oil, with a touch of garlic. Coleslaw mix and "brocco-slaw"—shredded broccoli stems—are good in stir-fries and skillet suppers.

- Precut veggies: Grab broccoli and cauliflower florets and celery sticks, add ranch dressing, and you've got the veggie thing covered. Put them in front of the kids and it may buy you enough time to actually cook something. At this writing, Trader Joe's, long a source of ready-to-steam fresh vegetables, has started carrying shredded cauliflower "rice" because of low-carb influence. And I rarely slice mushrooms anymore. Why bother when you can buy them that way?

- Bottled dressings: Skip low-fat dressings; most are full of corn syrup, and you're not eating a low-fat diet. Avoid sweet dressings like honey mustard, red "French," and poppy seed. Read labels!

- Sprinkle-on seasoning blends: These lend interest to the simple cuts of meat that are quickest and easiest to cook. My favorite go-to food is a pan-broiled pork shoulder steak with Tony Chachere's Creole Seasoning. I also love McCormick's Mediterranean Sea Salt Grinder; this is especially nice with lamb or poultry. Read labels; many seasoning blends contain sugar.

- Grocery store salad bar: Better than fast food! A few greens, a little green bell pepper and cucumber, plus shredded cheese, chopped hard-boiled egg, flaked tuna, chopped turkey breast or ham, crumbled bacon. The dressings are the treacherous part; see above. Look for olive oil and vinegar, along with salt and pepper. Salad bars are also great for precut vegetables.

- Frozen vegetables: More nutritious than canned, unless you plan to drink all the liquid in that can. Microwave according to package directions for best and quickest results. Steer clear of blends with pasta or other added carbs. Also skip varieties with sauces; they're likely to have hydrogenated oils, and very possibly sugars.

COOKING AHEAD

I am thinking of a conversation with a low-carb friend who told me that he'd been doing yard work over the weekend, so he fired up his smoker—he's a Kentucky boy—and smoked a couple of chickens and a big ol' pork shoulder. He and his wife had meat for the week.

My sister, a middle school science teacher, has for many years now spent an hour or two on Sunday afternoon making a double batch of soup or chili, and roasting a big hunk of meat—a double-batch meat loaf, a pork roast, a small turkey, or the like. These then serve her and her husband as lunch and supper for the rest of the week. She adds bagged salad or a quick steamed or grilled vegetable, and that's it.

Consider, too, deli-style salads—homemade coleslaw, UnPotato Salad (page 70), any salad you can make a vat of and pull out at a quarter-to-starvation. Make big batches of this sort of thing, especially if you have a family.

I recommend this approach wholeheartedly. Why cook just enough for one meal when you can, in the same time, cook enough for two or three? Leftovers are your friend.

A GOOD WORD
ABOUT FAST FOOD

Fast food is so often vilified, and so often deserves it, that it's nice to be able to say something happy about the industry. So here it is: Despite cries from activists about how fast-food places should be required to post nutritional information—usually demanding calorie counts—the fast-food industry has made more nutritional information available than virtually any other branch of the food service industry. Name a fast-food chain, and I will bet you a good steak dinner that they have a website that lists calories, carbs, fat, protein, etc. Many of them have calculators that let you subtract ingredients —e.g., "hold the bun." If you have questions, they will very likely have a customer service number. Further, many make nutritional information available in the store, either on a poster or in pamphlets, should you not have a smartphone at hand.

It is up to you to make use of this information.

WHAT ABOUT THE BUDGET?

There is no denying that many high-carb foods— noodles, rice, beans, potatoes—are cheap at the checkout. This is why they're staples of many budget-conscious families. How will low carb affect the bottom line?

First, know this: Any food that is making you fat, sick, and tired—that leads to escalating medical costs and very possibly to disability—would not be cheap if they were giving it away. There is a huge back-end payment on cheap, carb-heavy food, both in terms of your life and health, and also in cold, hard cash. You can't afford that cheap junk.

Not all carbs are cheap. I consider cold cereal to be a conspiracy to get suckers to pay 4 bucks for 15 cents' worth of grain. Stuff like microwave popcorn and potato chips are just ways to justify higher prices for low-cost commodities. Stop buying this junk and you'll free up dollars to spend on real food.

And real food comes in a wide range of prices. If you're flush you can eat rib-eye steaks, lobster dipped in lemon butter, and out-of-season asparagus every night, but you don't have to. You can eat dark-meat chicken quarters, pork shoulder, spareribs, and other inexpensive cuts.

Your body doesn't care whether your protein comes from pheasant or chicken, from lobster or tilapia, from prime rib or pork shoulder. It doesn't care if you eat radicchio or cabbage. It cares whether you give it the nutrients it needs, and that you don't feed it poison. Your cells have no idea what the price tag is, and they don't care.

Extra freezer and fridge space are valuable tools. If you can eke out the money and space for a deep freezer, even a little 5-cubic-foot chest freezer, do. It will save you money in the long run, stocking up at loss-leader sales.

Remember, too, you will be less hungry. If you're used to midafternoon munchies, to rummaging for a snack an hour after dinner, you will be shocked at just how much your appetite is reduced. At first you'll maintain some semblance of your customary eating patterns, but over time you may well discover that you're skipping snacks and automatically eating smaller portions at meals.

Do not force yourself to do this! If you're hungry, eat the unlimited protein-and-fat foods. Just know that over time your food bills may drop because you're simply not as hungry as you used to be.

A FEW INVALUABLE INGREDIENTS

Sweeteners

No matter what sweetener I use in a recipe, someone will object. Therefore, I am officially sidestepping the issue with this book. I am using:

- Granular sucralose (Splenda and knock-offs): The granular stuff is bulked with maltodextrin, a carbohydrate. Why does it say "0 carbs" on the package? Federal labeling law allows manufacturers to round down anything under 0.5 gram per serving. Accordingly, I count 0.5 gram of carb per teaspoon, or 24 grams per cup, and I use liquid sucralose instead when I can. The packets have less maltodextrin, so fewer carbs, but for more than a teaspoon or two of sugar's worth of sweetening, the packets are a pain. Do not use Splenda Sugar Blend or Brown Sugar Blend. As the names suggest, they contain sugar.

- Stevia in the Raw: Stevia in the Raw is stevia combined with maltodextrin, the same carbohydrate used to bulk Splenda, again, so that it measures like sugar. Figure about the same carb count as granular sucralose—0.5 gram per teaspoon, or 24 grams per cup. I use it only when a liquid sweetener will not do.

- Erythritol: A member of the polyol or sugar alcohol family, erythritol is technically a carbohydrate. However, unlike the other sugar alcohols, which are absorbed to varying degrees, erythritol is passed through the body unchanged. It does not raise blood sugar, and unlike most of the other sugar alcohols, it has little to no gastric effect.

  Erythritol comes with a couple of challenges: It is only 60 to 70 percent as sweet as sugar. It is also endothermic, meaning that when it hits the moisture in your mouth it absorbs energy and creates a cooling sensation—fine in ice cream, but disconcerting in a cookie. Because of these two properties, I often combine erythritol with liquid stevia extract. I generally start with half the erythritol, by volume, as the quantity of sugar called for in the original recipe. Then I add liquid stevia to bring it up to full sweetness. This works well.

  Look for erythritol at health food stores or online. Several brands are available from Amazon.com and Netrition.com; Amazon carries a few non-GMO versions if this concerns you.

  Because erythritol is neither digested nor absorbed, we have not included it in the carbohydrate counts for these recipes. Do not take this to mean that you can similarly discount the other sugar alcohol sweeteners.

- Liquid sucralose: I like EZ-Sweetz brand, available through Amazon.com or Netrition.com. You can get teeny bottles that fit nicely in a purse or pocket, to keep on hand for coffee. You need to know the sweetness equivalency of your liquid sucralose. The EZ-Sweetz I have on hand is the Family Size, and 1 drop equals 1 teaspoon of sugar. EZ-Sweetz Travel Size is twice as sweet—1 drop is the equivalent of 2 teaspoons of sugar. At the time of publication, the brand is offering free samples of the Travel Size strength at www.ez-sweetz.com/free-sample.

- Liquid stevia: I avoided stevia for a long time, finding the pure powdered extracts hard to use and unpleasantly bitter. The liquid extracts are far easier to use. I use NOW and SweetLeaf brands, both of which come in a wide variety of flavors. In these recipes you'll find vanilla, chocolate,

English toffee, and lemon drop flavored, along with plain—i.e., just sweet—liquid stevia. If your health food store doesn't carry these, they can very likely order them for you. You can also order these from Amazon.com.

Liquid stevia is far sweeter than sugar; it is important to know the sweetness equivalency. The NOW and SweetLeaf brands run roughly 6 drops equals 1 teaspoon of sugar, so 18 drops equals 1 tablespoon of sugar. I use ¼ teaspoon to replace ¼ cup of sugar, and ½ teaspoon to replace ½ cup of sugar. If you choose another brand, you'll need to check the label or their website for sweetness equivalency.

I have generally specified the sweetener I would be likely to use in a given recipe. However, if other sweeteners would work, I have listed them below the recipe under the heading "Alternative Sweetener." If no alternate sweetener is listed, it's because I am dubious about substitution.

Other Okay Sweeteners

Other HEAL-legal sweeteners include pure powdered stevia extract, Truvia, Monk Fruit in the Raw, Swerve, and Natural Mate. For ease of use, however, I have only included equivalencies for the above sweeteners. If you want to adapt recipes to use one of these other sweeteners, you'll need to learn the sweetness equivalency and do a little basic arithmetic.

Sweeteners Not Permitted

People search endlessly for a way around the no-sugar rule, so let me deter you by listing sweeteners that are not allowed:

- Agave nectar
- Coconut sugar
- Corn syrup, organic corn syrup
- Crystalline fructose
- Date sugar
- Honey
- Maple syrup
- Organic sugar, organic cane sugar
- Palm sugar
- Sucanat

All of these are out, for the simple reason that they're sugar.

I get queries about xylitol, which is popular in low-carb and paleo circles. Like erythritol, it is a member of the polyol or sugar alcohol family. However, according to a table in the Sugar Alcohol Fact Sheet at FoodInsight.org, we absorb xylitol at ten times the rate we do erythritol. This makes erythritol the clear choice.

Xanthan and Guar

These are finely milled soluble fibers, which are hugely useful in low-carb cuisine. Use in place of flour, cornstarch, or arrowroot for thickening sauces or soups. What do they taste like? Nothing at all; they couldn't be blander.

They are powerful thickeners, so do not try a one-for-one substitution. The results could be used to surface roads. Fill an old salt or spice shaker with whichever you have on hand—I marginally prefer xanthan—and keep it by the stove. When you have a sauce or soup you need to thicken, start whisking first, then *lightly* sprinkle the thickener over the surface as you whisk. Go slowly; it's easy to put in more and impossible to remove too much. Keep in mind that these continue to thicken a bit on standing, so quit when your dish is a little less thick than you want it to be.

Both of these thickeners will keep pretty much forever as long as they're dry.

These also lend structure to nut- or seed-meal–based baked goods. I've used them in a few recipes to improve texture.

Again, these are health food store items, and again, they can be ordered online, too.

Shirataki Noodles

Most "low-carb" noodles are nothing I'll eat. One widely distributed brand, made with the same ingredients as standard pasta, wound up paying reparations to consumers they'd fooled. The only noodles I eat are shirataki, and they are a staple in my kitchen.

Shirataki are traditional Japanese noodles made from the fiber glucomannan, derived from *konjac* or *konnyaku*, a root vegetable. (This is often translated as "yam.") Made almost entirely of fiber, shirataki are very low in both carbohydrate and calories.

Shirataki come in two basic varieties: traditional and tofu. Traditional shirataki are made entirely of glucomannan fiber. They're translucent and gelatinous, quite different from the wheat-based noodles we grew up on. I only like them in Asian recipes— sesame noodles, Asian soups, and the like.

Tofu shirataki, as the name suggests, have a little bit of tofu added to the glucomannan. This makes them white, and more tender than traditional shirataki. They're not identical to regular pasta, but they're closer, and I like them in all sorts of things, from fettuccine Alfredo to tuna casserole. Both kinds come in a variety of widths and shapes.

Shirataki come prehydrated in a pouch of liquid. To use them, snip open the pouch and dump them into a strainer in the sink. You'll notice the liquid smells fishy. Do not panic. Rinse your noodles well, and put them in a microwavable bowl. Nuke them on high for 2 minutes, and drain them again. Nuke them for *another* 2 minutes, and drain them one more time. This renders them quite bland, and cooks out extra liquid that would otherwise dilute sauces.

Long noodles are considered good luck in Japan, but I find shirataki a bit too long. I snip across them a few times with my kitchen shears. All of this microwaving and draining and snipping takes less time than boiling water for standard pasta.

You now have hot noodles! Add sauce, stir them into soup, or do whatever you like to do with noodles.

I can get shirataki at my local health food stores and Asian markets. You can order them online, but be aware: They do not tolerate freezing; they disintegrate into mush. This means you may not want to order them in the dead of winter. But they keep for months in the fridge, so if you decide you like them, go ahead and stock up.

Whey Protein Powder

A few of these recipes call for vanilla or chocolate whey protein powder. I've used several brands over the years, and never had one not work. The Designer Protein brand is perhaps most widely available; GNC stores carry it. Recently I've been using Vitacost.com's house brand, because the price is right, and it's fine. Need I remind you to read labels or online nutrition info to be sure there's no sugar?

Protein powder is sold in canisters that hold a pound or more. As long as you store them tightly closed and in a dry place, they should keep for a long, long time.

Bouillon Concentrate

I use bouillon concentrate as a seasoning. My preferred form is Better Than Bouillon Base. It actually contains some of the protein source listed on the label and is gluten-free; I think the flavor is superior to granules or cubes. I keep their beef and chicken pastes on hand.

Vege-Sal

One of my favorite seasonings, Vege-Sal is a blend of salt and powdered vegetables. It's subtle, but I think it improves many savory dishes, and you'll see that I often have specified "salt or Vege-Sal."

Vege-Sal is made by Modern Products, and has recently had their popular "Spike" name added to the title, so it's Spike Vege-Sal. If your health food store doesn't have it, they can order it for you, or you can order it online. Or just use salt.

If you're going to try Vege-Sal, be aware that along with coming in a shaker, you can buy it in 10- or 20-ounce (280 or 560 g) boxes. If you decide you like it, this is considerably cheaper than buying a shaker every time you need Vege-Sal!

Sugar-Free Coffee Flavoring Syrup

A few recipes in this book call for sugar-free coffee flavoring syrup. I've tried sugar-free varieties from DaVinci Gourmet, Torani, and Monin, and like them all. Check grocery stores and coffee shops, but like everything else, if you can't find them locally, you can order them online.

Sriracha

This hot sauce is taking over the world. A specialty ingredient a decade ago, it is now everywhere. The original Huy Fong brand, with the rooster on the label, contains a little sugar. I have discovered Dark Star brand, which does not. I get it at Bloomingfoods, my local health food co-op, or you can order it from Amazon.com.

CHAPTER 3
Snacks and Other Finger Foods

Around the middle of the twentieth century, Americans got sold, first on the idea of snacks—that we needed to eat between meals—and then on the notion that "snack" properly meant something crunchy and salty in a cellophane bag. The idea of watching a movie or spending a night playing board games without munchies seems wrong, somehow.

There is one type of food that a low-carb diet doesn't include: Stuff that can be eaten endlessly, mindlessly, through a two-hour movie or an evening of binge watching. Unlike carb-heavy snacks—potato chips, pretzels, popcorn, and the like—low-carb foods fill you up. Protein and fat trigger satiety. Overeat and you may well make yourself sick.

Let me plant this thought in your mind: As you grow used to eating this way, experiencing stable blood sugar and eating filling meals of protein and fat, your need for and interest in snacks may well fade. You won't have blood sugar crashes driving you to eat something, anything, to get it back up again. Take pleasure in the luxurious food you are allowed, and in the utter lack of hunger a low-carb diet brings. If you're hungry, eat. If you're hungry between meals, eat something from this chapter.

My favorite use for these finger foods is as an alternative to a traditional meal. It's family movie night? Skip the full meal routine. Instead, put out a few of these tempting and filling finger foods, and let everyone nibble.

Most of these make fabulous party foods, too. The word "diet" will not cross your guests' minds.

1 slice American cheese—the deluxe stuff

YIELD: 1 serving
70 calories; 6 g fat; 4 g protein; 0 g carbohydrate; 0 g dietary fiber per serving

CHEESE CRACKERS

You can do this with "real"—i.e., unprocessed—cheese, and it will come out crisp and delicious. But there's something about the deluxe processed American that puffs up in a remarkably cracker-y way.

Coat a microwavable plate with nonstick cooking spray, and lay the cheese on it. Microwave for 60 to 75 seconds. Let it cool a minute or so, peel it off the plate, and eat. If you'd like more cracker-y-size crackers, cut the cheese into quarters before you nuke it.

1 cup (115 g) shredded Cheddar cheese—with no additives

½ teaspoon garlic powder

½ teaspoon onion powder

¼ teaspoon cayenne, or to taste

YIELD: 4 servings
116 calories; 9 g fat; 7 g protein; 1 g carbohydrate; trace dietary fiber per serving

NACHO CHEESE CRISPS

Here we have proof that the flavor of processed snack foods does not lie in the carbs. Cheesy-spicy-crunchy good!

Put the shredded cheese in a bowl and sprinkle the seasonings over the top, tossing as you go.

Coat a microwavable plate with nonstick cooking spray—I used a salad-size plate. Put about ¼ cup (30 g) of cheese on the plate, and nuke on high for 2 to 3 minutes, or until you've got a crispy disk that looks sort of like an orange surface of the moon. Let it cool a minute or two, loosen it from the surface of the plate by sliding a knife underneath, and cook another batch. I had to respray the plate between batches.

1 ounce (28 g) pepperoni slices

YIELD: 1 serving

141 calories; 12 g fat; 6 g protein;
1 g carbohydrate; 0 g dietary fiber
per serving

Chicken skin—however much
you have on hand

Salt, to taste

PEPPERONI CHIPS

Got a crunchy craving? I love these pepperoni chips! Dip them in whipped cream cheese. They'd be good crumbled over a salad, too.

Lay your pepperoni slices on a microwavable plate, and nuke them for 60 to 90 seconds, or until crisp. That is all.

CHICKEN CHIPS

Every time I mention Chicken Chips online I get demands for the recipe. As you can see, it's super-simple. If you love crispy chicken skin, this is the ultimate low-carb snack.

Preheat oven to 350ºF (180ºC, or gas mark 4). Spread your chicken skin flat on your broiler rack. Throw in any chunks of fat, too. Bake them until they're brown and crisp, at least 20 minutes. Season them with salt to taste.

I have no way of knowing the exact nutrition count on these, since I can't find a listing for just chicken skin. Nor do I know how much of the fat in them cooks out, exactly. I know they're high in fat, and also in gelatin, which is very good stuff. I have my local specialty butcher shop save me 10 pounds (4.5 kg) or so of skin at a time. (Here's a shout-out to the Butcher's Block in Bloomington, Indiana—you guys rock!) Then I freeze it in sandwich-size resealable plastic bags; they hold just about enough to cover the broiler rack.

Don't forget to pour the rendered chicken fat into a jar for cooking! That's schmaltz, one of the most beloved fats in Jewish cuisine.

3 tablespoons (45 g) butter

2 to 3 tablespoons (30 to 45 g) powdered erythritol*

¼ teaspoon ground cinnamon

3½ ounces (100 g) plain pork rinds or skins

***Alternative Sweeteners**

2 to 3 tablespoons (3 to 4.5 g) Splenda

2 to 3 tablespoons (6 to 9 g) Stevia in the Raw

YIELD: 5 servings
169 calories; 13 g fat; 12 g protein; trace carbohydrate; trace dietary fiber per serving

BUTTER-CINNAMON CRISPIES

For everyone who misses cinnamon graham crackers, cinnamon rolls—cinnamon anything. I know it sounds odd, but try these. They really are remarkably good.

Preheat oven to 350°F (180°C, or gas mark 4). While it's heating, put the butter in a roasting pan and put it in the oven to melt.

In a small dish, mix together the powdered erythritol and cinnamon.

When the butter is melted, dump the pork rinds into the pan, and toss till they're all evenly covered with butter—this takes a bit of persistence.

Sprinkle the erythritol-cinnamon mixture over the pork rinds, stirring the whole time, so as to get it as evenly distributed as possible.

Slide the pan into the oven, and give it 5 minutes. Pull it out and stir again. Give it another 5, and they're done.

2 tablespoons (30 g) coconut oil

2 cups (200 g) pecan halves

1 tablespoon (9 g) Creole seasoning (I like Tony Chachere's More Spice Seasoning)

YIELD: 8 servings
213 calories; 22 g fat; 2 g protein; 6 g carbohydrate; 2 g dietary fiber per serving

CAJUN PECANS

Super-easy, super-addictive. Your biggest challenge will be sticking to the ¼-cup (55 g) serving size. You might want to make single-serving bags and stash them out of sight.

Preheat oven to 350°F (180°C, or gas mark 4). While it's heating, put the coconut oil in a roasting pan, and stick it in the oven for a few minutes to melt.

When the oil has melted, dump your pecans into the pan, and stir till they're all coated. Now spread evenly, and put them back in the oven. Give them 10 minutes.

Pull them out of the oven, stir in the Creole seasoning, and let them cool. Store in an airtight container.

2½ tablespoons (35 g) coconut oil

2 teaspoons (2 g) ground rosemary

¼ teaspoon cayenne

2 cups (200 g) walnuts

Salt, to taste

YIELD: 8 servings

227 calories; 22 g fat; 8 g protein; 4 g carbohydrate; 2 g dietary fiber per serving

ROSEMARY WALNUTS

Subtle but dazzling. I've given away little tins of these for Christmas, and people loved them.

Preheat oven to 300ºF (150ºC, or gas mark 2).

While the oven is heating, put the coconut oil in a roasting pan, and put it in the oven. Give it a few minutes to melt the oil.

When the oil is melted, pull out the pan and measure the rosemary and cayenne into the pan. Stir them into the coconut oil until they're evenly distributed.

Now add the walnuts to the pan. Stir very well, making sure they're all evenly coated with the seasoned oil, then spread them in an oven layer Put the pan back in the oven, and set your timer for 5 minutes.

When the timer beeps, stir your walnuts well—I used a rubber scraper, and scraped the seasoned oil up off the bottom of the pan as I stirred, to work it into the walnuts better. Again, spread in an even layer, and put them back in the oven. Set your timer for another 5 minutes.

Repeat the stirring, and put them back for 5 more minutes. Then cool, season with salt to taste, and store in an airtight container.

4 pounds (1.8 kg) chicken wings

1 cup (100 g) grated Parmesan cheese (use the cheap stuff in the green shaker)

2 tablespoons (2.5 g) dried parsley

1 tablespoon (3 g) dried oregano

2 teaspoons (5 g) paprika

1 teaspoon salt

½ teaspoon ground black pepper

½ cup (112 g) butter

YIELD: About 50 pieces

68 calories; 5 g fat; 4 g protein; trace carbohydrate; trace dietary fiber per piece

WICKED WINGS

These wings are utterly, totally addictive! They're a bit messy and time-consuming to make, but worth every minute. They'll impress the heck out of your friends, too, and you'll wish you'd made more of them. They also taste great the next day.

This is one of the most popular (and most pirated) recipes I've ever published. The one criticism I see is that they're too salty. If you tend to like things less salty, cut the salt to ½ teaspoon. Feel free to use this cheese mixture on thighs or breasts, too.

Preheat oven to 350°F (180°C, or gas mark 4). Line a shallow baking pan with foil. (Do not omit this step, or you'll still be scrubbing the pan a week later.)

Cut the wings into single joints, saving the pointy tips for broth. Or not. Up to you.

Combine the Parmesan cheese and the parsley, oregano, paprika, salt, and pepper in a bowl.

Melt the butter in a shallow bowl or pan.

Dip each wing joint in butter, roll in the cheese-and-seasoning mixture, and arrange in the foil-lined pan.

Bake for 1 hour—and then kick yourself for not having made a double recipe!

3 cloves garlic, minced very fine

1 tablespoon (15 ml) olive oil

8 large chicken wings, whole, not cut into drumettes

1 tablespoon (7 g) paprika

1 teaspoon dried oregano

1 teaspoon salt

1 teaspoon ground black pepper

¼ teaspoon cayenne

1 lime, cut into wedges

YIELD: 4 servings

264 calories; 19 g fat; 19 g protein; 4 g carbohydrate; 1 g dietary fiber per serving

SPICY SPANISH WINGS

These are so good that our tester Kelly was considering a serious relationship with them. Super-simple, too, and a nice change from the usual Buffalo wings. You can play with this by using different kinds of paprika—hot if you're a chili-head, sweet if you're not, even smoked paprika for an extra kick.

Mix the garlic with the olive oil, and let them sit together for at least 10 minutes, to let the flavor of the garlic infuse the oil. Then brush the wings all over with the oil.

Meanwhile, preheat a grill or broiler.

In a large bowl, combine the paprika, oregano, salt, pepper, and cayenne, and mix them well. Add the wings, and toss to coat.

Grill or broil the wings for about 15 minutes—you want them done through, with a crispy skin and a few blackened spots. Serve with lime wedges to squeeze over them.

12 hard-boiled eggs

⅔ cup (150 g) mayonnaise

1 tablespoon (11 g) brown mustard

1 teaspoon Tabasco sauce, or other Louisiana-style hot sauce

Salt and ground black pepper, to taste

Paprika

YIELD: 24 servings (1 half)

83 calories; 8 g fat; 3 g protein; trace carbohydrate; trace dietary fiber per serving

DEVILED EGGS

Deviled eggs are hugely popular for parties. They're old-fashioned, yet every time I show up with a platter of them, people say, "Oh! Deviled eggs!" They're also great to have waiting in the fridge when you come home hungry. A couple of halves, and you'll be full for hours.

Peel the eggs, turning the yolks out into your food processor. Yes, I have started using my food processor to mix deviled eggs; it makes them incomparably creamy. Set the whites on a platter or in a big, flat snap-top container, if you're planning to store or transport them.

Add the mayonnaise, mustard, and Tabasco to the yolks. Run the processor, scraping down the sides a few times, until the mixture is completely creamy. Season with salt and pepper to taste.

Now stuff the yolks into the whites. I like to spoon the yolks into my pastry bag and pipe them in using a star tip, but a spoon works just fine.

Sprinkle with paprika, and serve or refrigerate.

12 hard-boiled eggs

¼ cup (60 g) mayonnaise

¼ cup (60 g) sour cream

½ cup (100 g) moist smoked salmon, mashed fine

2 tablespoons (30 g) jarred, grated horseradish

4 teaspoons (13 g) finely minced sweet red onion

¼ teaspoon salt

YIELD: 24 servings (1 half)
129 calories; 10 g fat; 8 g protein; 1 g carbohydrate; trace dietary fiber per serving

FISH EGGS

That's eggs with fish, not eggs from fish. If you thought stuffed eggs couldn't go to an upscale party, these will change your mind.

Slice the eggs in half and carefully remove the yolks into a mixing bowl.

Mash the yolks with a fork. Stir in the mayonnaise, sour cream, salmon, horseradish, onion, and salt, and mix until creamy.

Spoon the mixture back into the hollows in the egg whites.

1 pound (455 g) fresh mushrooms

1 can (6 ounces, or 170 g) crabmeat

2 ounces (60 g) cream cheese

¼ cup (60 g) mayonnaise

¼ cup (25 g) grated Parmesan cheese

12 scallions, minced

¼ teaspoon ground black pepper

1 dash Tabasco sauce

YIELD: 25 servings (1 piece)
41 calories; 3 g fat; 3 g protein; 1 g carbohydrate; trace dietary fiber per serving

KAY'S CRAB-STUFFED MUSHROOMS

My friend Kay begged me to come up with low-carb crab puffs. I tried several different approaches, but, alas, they eluded me. So I came up with these mushrooms instead, and she loved them.

Preheat oven to 325ºF (170ºC, or gas mark 3).

Wipe the mushrooms clean with a damp cloth, and remove the stems.

In a mixing bowl, combine the crab, cream cheese, mayonnaise, Parmesan, scallions, pepper, and Tabasco, mixing well. Spoon the mixture into the mushroom caps, and arrange them in a large, flat roasting pan.

Bake for 45 minutes to 1 hour, or until the mushrooms are done through. Serve hot.

6 small portobello mushrooms, totaling 6 ounces (170 g)

1 package (6 ounces, or 170 g) garlic-and-herb spreadable cheese (such as Boursin or Alouette)

2 tablespoons (10 g) crushed plain pork rinds or skins

YIELD: 6 servings
120 calories; 12 g fat; 2 g protein; 2 g carbohydrate; trace dietary fiber per serving

1½ pounds (680 g) mushrooms

2 tablespoons (28 g) butter

½ cup (80 g) chopped onion

4 cloves garlic, crushed

1 package (10 ounces, or 280 g) frozen chopped spinach, thawed

4 ounces (115 g) cream cheese

¼ cup (25 g) Parmesan cheese, plus a little extra for sprinkling

1½ teaspoons Worcestershire sauce

½ teaspoon salt or Vege-Sal

¼ teaspoon ground black pepper

YIELD: 40 servings (1 piece)
24 calories; 2 g fat; 1 g protein; 1 g carbohydrate; trace dietary fiber per serving

GARLIC-CHEESE STUFFED MUSHROOMS

These are the easiest stuffed mushrooms you'll ever make, and they're really yummy, too. Feel free to use good old button mushrooms, if you prefer.

Preheat oven to 350°F (180°C, or gas mark 4).

Wipe the mushrooms clean and remove the stems (save them to slice and sauté to serve over steaks or in omelets). Divide the cheese between the mushroom caps. Sprinkle each one with a teaspoon of pork rind crumbs.

Arrange the mushrooms in a shallow baking pan. Add just enough water to film the bottom of the pan. Bake for 30 minutes and serve hot.

SPINACH STUFFED MUSHROOMS

I took these to my Toastmasters Christmas party. People scarfed them right down!

Preheat oven to 350°F (180°C, or gas mark 4).

Wipe the mushrooms clean and remove the stems. Set the caps aside and chop the stems fairly fine.

In a large, heavy skillet, over medium-low heat, melt the butter. Add the chopped stems and the onion. Sauté these until the mushroom bits are changing color and the onion is soft and translucent. Add the garlic, stir it up, and sauté for another couple of minutes.

While that's happening, dump your thawed spinach into a strainer and press all the water out of it that you can. Now stir it into the mushroom-onion mixture. Next, stir in the cream cheese. When it's melted, add the Parmesan cheese, Worcestershire sauce, salt, and pepper.

Stuff the spinach-mushroom mixture into the mushroom caps. Arrange the stuffed caps in a baking pan as you stuff them.

When they're all stuffed, sprinkle a little Parmesan cheese over them to make them look nice. Add enough water to just barely cover the bottom of the pan. Bake for 30 minutes. Serve warm.

CHAPTER 4
A Few Grain Substitutes

There is no actual grain in this chapter, but you'll find some comforting substitutes.

These recipes are some of the most complex in the book, for a simple reason: Baking is the most complicated form of cooking, and adapting starchy, sugary baking recipes to low carb makes them, if anything, even more complex. What's more, many of the ingredients commonly used in low-carb baked goods are still too high in carbs for the HEAL Protocol.

I have searched my archives carefully to find these recipes, and have even come up with a few new ones. I hope you enjoy them. Just be careful to keep an eye on those portion sizes!

7 ounces (200 g) plain pork rinds or skins

½ cup (112 g) butter

½ teaspoon liquid stevia (English toffee)

¼ teaspoon corn flavoring (optional)

1 cup (240 g) erythritol

YIELD: 8 servings

237 calories; 19 g fat; 15 g protein; trace carbohydrate; 0 g dietary fiber per serving

QUORK

Remember Quisp and Quake, not to mention Cap'n Crunch? This is the pork rind equivalent, and it's insanely good. You can eat it plain, of course, or just like cereal, with your 3 tablespoons (45 ml) of heavy cream, or with carb-reduced milk or sugar-free almond milk. It's also a great substitute for caramel corn. Both LorAnn and Amoretti make corn flavoring, both in buttered popcorn and sweet corn. Either will work here. I got mine through Amazon.com.

Preheat oven to 275ºF (130ºC). While it's heating, break your pork rinds up into bits about the size of cold cereal.

When the oven is hot, put the butter in your biggest roasting pan and put it in the oven to melt.

When the butter is melted, pull the pan out of the oven. Add the liquid stevia and corn flavoring, if using. Stir them into the butter.

Add the pork rinds to the pan, and, using a pancake turner, stir them into the butter until they're all evenly coated.

Sprinkle the erythritol over the pork rinds ¼ cup (60 g) at a time, stirring each addition in well before adding more.

When all the erythritol is worked in, slide the pan back into the oven. Toast the pork rinds for 40 minutes, stirring everything very well with a pancake turner every 10 minutes.

At the end of 40 minutes, remove from the oven and let your Quork cool in the pan before storing in an airtight container.

3½ ounces (100 g) plain pork rinds or skins (There are bags that hold 3½ ounces.)

1 teaspoon ground cinnamon

½ teaspoon baking powder

4 eggs

½ cup (120 ml) heavy cream

¼ teaspoon liquid stevia (English toffee), or more to taste*

Water, as needed

3 tablespoons (45 g) butter, plus more for serving

---

*Alternative Sweetener

3 tablespoons (45 ml) caramel sugar-free coffee flavoring syrup

---

YIELD: 3 servings
(3 pancakes per serving)
508 calories; 42 g fat; 29 g protein; 3 g carbohydrate; trace dietary fiber per serving

SALTED CARAMEL–CINNAMON PANCAKES

Here is where you will assume I have slipped a cog, gone 'round the bend, flat-out low-carb crackers. Pork rind pancakes? Yes, my friends, and a thing of wonder they are, somewhere between pancakes and French toast. You simply must try this. You will be amazed. If you prefer, you can cook these in your waffle iron instead. Yum.

Run the pork rinds through your food processor till you have fine crumbs. Dump 'em in a mixing bowl.

Add the cinnamon and baking powder, and stir 'em into the crumbs.

In a separate bowl, whisk together the eggs, cream, and stevia. Pour this into the crumbs, and whisk till everything's evenly wet.

Let this mixture sit for 5 minutes or so. This would be a good time to put your frying pan or griddle over medium heat; you'll want it hot when the batter is ready.

Okay, come back to your batter. It will have been thick to start with, and will have thickened even more on standing, becoming downright gloppy. Thin it with water to a consistency you like—I keep mine pretty thick so I get ½-inch (1 cm) thick pancakes.

Melt half of the butter in your skillet or on the griddle, and start frying your pancakes like you would any pancakes. Let them get nicely browned on the first side before flipping and cooking the other. The rest of the butter is for the second round, of course.

Serve with more butter and a sprinkle of Cinnamon "Sugar" (page 160).

3½ ounces (100 g) plain pork rinds or skins

¼ cup (60 g) erythritol*

¼ cup (32 g) vanilla whey protein powder

¼ cup (28 g) almond meal

½ teaspoon baking powder

¼ teaspoon ground cinnamon

5 eggs

1½ cups (355 ml) water

---

*Alternative Sweeteners

¼ teaspoon liquid stevia

12 drops EZ-Sweetz Family Size

6 drops EZ-Sweetz Travel Size

YIELD: 12 servings (1 waffle)
103 calories; 5 g fat; 12 g protein; 2 g carbohydrate; trace dietary fiber per serving

PORK RIND WAFFLES

I was determined to give you waffles! I tried several recipes that didn't cut it—limp and tasting only of eggs. These worked out! And geez, are they filling. What with whipping the egg whites and all, you'll want to make these over the weekend. Reheat in the toaster or toaster oven for a grab-and-go breakfast.

Plug in your waffle iron. You want it hot when the batter is ready.

Run the pork rinds through your food processor until they're powdered. Dump the pork rind crumbs into a mixing bowl.

Add the erythritol, protein powder, almond meal, baking powder, and cinnamon. Use a whisk to stir everything together well.

Separate the eggs, putting the whites into a deep, narrow mixing bowl and the yolks in with the pork rind mixture. Since the tiniest speck of yolk will keep your egg whites from whipping, do yourself a favor and separate each one into a custard cup first.

Whisk the egg yolks and the water into the pork rind mixture. Let this sit while you do the next step.

Using an electric mixer, whip the egg whites until they stand in stiff peaks.

With a rubber scraper, gently fold the egg whites into the pork rind mixture, adding one-quarter of the whites and incorporating them well before adding another quarter, and so on.

Bake the batter according to the instructions that come with your waffle iron.

Serve immediately, with butter and Cinnamon "Sugar" (page 160) or Maple Butter (page 160).

To freeze, cool on paper towels to absorb moisture, then put in resealable plastic bags with the towels still between them. Reheat in the toaster or toaster oven, rather than the microwave, so your waffles will be crisp.

4 eggs

1 cup (250 g) ricotta cheese

½ cup (64 g) vanilla whey protein powder

1 teaspoon baking powder

¼ teaspoon salt

2 tablespoons (28 g) butter

YIELD: 30 silver dollar pancakes
45 calories; 3 g fat; 5 g protein; 1 g carbohydrate; trace dietary fiber per pancake

(If you eat 6 of these silver dollar pancakes, you'll get 268 calories, 16 g fat, 27 g protein, 4 g carbohydrate, and 1 g fiber.)

PERFECT PROTEIN PANCAKES

These taste just like mom used to make; you'd never guess they were low carb. Make extras over the weekend for quick breakfasts on busy mornings.

Coat a heavy skillet or griddle with nonstick cooking spray and place it over medium heat.

In a mixing bowl, whisk together the eggs and ricotta until quite smooth. Whisk in the protein powder, baking powder, and salt, only mixing until well combined.

Melt 1 tablespoon (14 g) of the butter on the hot skillet or griddle, and drop batter onto it by the tablespoonful. When the bubbles on the surface of the pancakes are breaking and leaving little holes around the edges, flip them and cook the other side.

Add the rest of the butter to cook the rest of the batter.

Serve these with Maple Butter (page 160) or Cinnamon "Sugar" (page 160).

---

4 eggs

½ cup (125 g) ricotta cheese

¼ cup (60 ml) heavy cream

36 drops liquid stevia*

½ teaspoon ground cinnamon

¼ teaspoon ground nutmeg

6 drops corn flavoring (optional)

1 teaspoon oil—I used MCT oil, but melted coconut oil would be fine

---

*Alternative Sweeteners

12 drops EZ-Sweetz Family Size

6 drops EZ-Sweetz Travel Size

YIELD: 4 servings
232 calories; 21 g fat; 9 g protein; 2 g carbohydrate; trace dietary fiber per serving

FRIED MUSH

Lightly adapted from a recipe my friend Diana Lee allowed me to use in *500 Low Carb Recipes*. Great for those of you who are tired of eggs. In the interest of full disclosure, I must tell you that as an unregenerate Yankee I have never had real fried cornmeal mush. But Diana has, and she vouches for this. It's really tasty regardless. LorAnn and Amoretti both make corn flavoring, in sweet and popcorn flavors. I got mine at Amazon.com.

Preheat oven to 350°F (180°C, or gas mark 4). Coat an 8-inch (20 cm) square baking dish with nonstick cooking spray.

Simply put everything but the oil in a mixing bowl. Whisk together, and pour into the prepared baking dish.

Bake for 25 minutes, or until a knife inserted in the center comes out clean. Pull it out of the oven and let it cool a few minutes.

Put your large, heavy skillet over medium heat, and add the oil. Cut the mush into 4 squares, and fry until they're golden on both sides. Serve with Cinnamon "Sugar" (page 160)

4 cups (340 g) shredded coconut meat

¾ cup (84 g) flaxseed meal

1 tablespoon (12 g) xanthan or guar

1 teaspoon erythritol—not essential, but I think it improves the flavor

1½ teaspoons baking soda

½ teaspoon salt

½ cup (120 ml) water

2 tablespoons (28 ml) cider vinegar

4 eggs

YIELD: 20 servings

111 calories; 9 g fat; 4 g protein; 5 g carbohydrate; 4 g dietary fiber per serving

COCONUT FLAX BREAD

This takes a decent food processor, but it's delicious and satisfying. Toast and spread with butter, or make an open-faced grilled cheese! This recipe first appeared in *The Fat Fast Cookbook*, which I wrote for CarbSmart. Thanks to my dear friend Andrew DiMino, who kindly granted permission for me to share it here.

Preheat oven to 350ºF (180ºC, or gas mark 4). Grease a loaf pan—standard, not super-huge; the opening on mine is 8½ × 4½ inches (26 × 11 cm). Now line it with nonstick aluminum foil or baking parchment.

In your food processor, with the S-blade in place, combine the coconut flaxseed meal, xanthan, erythritol, baking soda, and salt. Run the processor till everything is ground to a fine meal. Scrape down the sides and run the processor some more.

While that's happening, in a glass measuring cup, combine the water and the vinegar. Have this standing by the food processor.

While the food processor is running, add the eggs, one at a time, through the feed tube.

Finally, pour the water-and-vinegar mixture in through the feed tube. Run just another 30 seconds or so.

Pour or scrape the batter into the prepared loaf pan. Bake for 1 hour and 15 minutes. Turn out onto a wire rack to cool.

This slices beautifully. I get 20 slices per loaf; don't slice extra thick or you'll be over your 5-gram limit. Do keep this refrigerated, or, better yet, slice it as soon as it's cool, then freeze.

1 cup (145 g) sunflower seed kernels

½ cup (80 g) rice protein powder (Nutribiotic makes this—ask at your health food store)

½ teaspoon xanthan or guar

½ teaspoon baking powder

½ teaspoon salt, plus more for sprinkling

2 tablespoons (28 g) butter, at room temperature

1½ tablespoons (1 g) minced fresh rosemary

1 cup (115 g) shredded sharp Cheddar cheese

½ cup (40 g) shredded Parmesan cheese

1 egg white

3 tablespoons (45 ml) water

YIELD: 50 servings (1 cracker)
42 calories; 3 g fat; 3 g protein; 1 g carbohydrate; trace dietary fiber per serving

ROSEMARY CHEESE CRACKERS

I saw a recipe for Rosemary Cheese Crackers, and while I wasn't going to use flour and stuff, the flavor combination sounded great. It is! These may be the best crackers I've ever done.

Preheat oven to 350°F (180°C, or gas mark 4).

Put the sunflower seeds, rice protein powder, xanthan or guar, baking powder, and salt in your food processor, and run till the sunflower seeds are ground up to the texture of cornmeal or finer.

With the processor running, add the butter and the rosemary. Then work in the cheeses in 3 or 4 additions.

With the processor still running, add the egg white, then the water. When you have a soft dough, turn off the processor.

Line a cookie sheet with baking parchment. Make a ball of half the dough, and put it on the parchment, then put another sheet of parchment over it.

Use your rolling pin to roll the dough out into as thin and even a sheet as you can. Carefully peel off the top sheet of parchment.

Use a straight, thin-bladed knife to score the dough into crackers—I make mine about the size of Wheat Thins. Sprinkle them lightly with salt.

Bake for 20 to 25 minutes, or until golden. Score again before removing from the parchment.

CHAPTER 5
Eggs and Cheese

Time to shift mental gears: Eggs are good for you. You can eat them daily. Furthermore, the yolk is by far the most nutritious part of the egg. Throw away yolks and you'll toss out all the vitamins, minerals, and antioxidants. If you love fried eggs over easy, with gooey, runny yolks, or soft-boiled eggs with butter melted into them, dig in!

(An idea that's not quite a recipe: I often top warmed-up leftovers with fried eggs to give them new appeal. I find fried eggs improve meat loaf, leftover hot vegetable dishes, whatever.)

Add to this that eggs are comparatively inexpensive, and quick and easy to cook, and you've got a low-carb superfood. And, as this chapter will demonstrate, they are endlessly variable. Have fun, and feel free to serve eggs not only for breakfast, but also for lunch and dinner.

As for cheese, quit with the low-fat stuff already; 1 to 2 ounces (28 to 55 g) of cheese per day will add terrific flavor and nutritional value to your menu. And don't miss the Backwards Pizza recipe (page 66) at the end of this chapter—the crust is made out of, you guessed it, cheese!

I'm assuming you already know how to fry, scramble, and boil eggs; I'm jumping right to something a little more complex.

DANA'S EASY OMELET METHOD

If I had to choose just one skill to teach to every new low-carber, it would be how to make an omelet. They're fast, they're easy, and they make a wide variety of simple ingredients seem like a meal.

You'll need a good pan: 9 to 10 inches (23 to 25 cm) in diameter, with sloping sides. Nonstick is preferable. If you've been leery of the chemicals used in traditional coatings, take a look at the new ceramic nonstick cookware. It's wonderful.

Have your filling ready. If you're using vegetables, you'll want to sauté them first. If you're using cheese, have it grated or sliced and ready to go. If you're making an omelet to use up leftovers—a great idea, by the way—warm them through in the microwave and have them standing by.

Coat your omelet pan well with cooking spray if it doesn't have a good nonstick surface, and put it over medium-high heat. While the skillet is heating, grab your eggs—two is the perfect number for this size pan, but one or three will work—and a bowl, crack the eggs, and beat them with a fork. Don't add any water or milk or anything, just mix them up.

The pan is hot enough when a drop of water thrown in sizzles instantly. Add the oil or butter, swirl it around to cover the bottom, then pour in the eggs all at once. They should sizzle, too, and immediately start to set. When the bottom layer of egg is set around the edges—this should happen quite quickly—lift the edge using a spatula and tip the pan to let the raw egg flow underneath. Do this all around the edges, until there's not enough raw egg to run.

Now, turn your burner to the lowest heat if you have a gas stove. If you have an electric stove, you'll need a "warm" burner standing by; electric elements don't cool off fast enough for this job. Put your filling on one half of the omelet, cover it, and let it sit over very low heat for a minute or two, no more. Peek and see if the raw, shiny egg is gone from the top surface (although you can serve it that way if you like—that's how the French prefer their omelets), and the cheese, if you've used some, is melted. If not, re-cover the pan and let it go another minute or two.

When your omelet is done, slip a spatula under the half without the filling and fold it over; then lift the whole thing onto a plate. Or you can get fancy and tip the pan, letting the filling side of the omelet slide onto the plate, folding the top over as you go, but this takes some practice.

This makes a single-serving omelet. I think it's easier to make several individual omelets than to make one big one, and omelets are so quick to make that it's not a big deal. Anyway, that way you can customize your omelets to each individual's taste. If you're making more than two or three omelets, keep them warm in your oven, set to its very lowest heat.

Now here are some ideas for what to put in your omelets!

2 eggs, beaten

2 teaspoons butter

1 ounce (28 g) Monterey Jack, pepper Jack, or Cheddar cheese, sliced or shredded

½ avocado, sliced

YIELD: 1 serving

372 calories; 32 g fat; 19 g protein; 7 g carbohydrate; 3 g dietary fiber per serving

MONTEREY JACK AND AVOCADO OMELET

The cheese and avocado combination is my favorite omelet. Avocados are so good for you—loaded with the healthiest of fats, and the best-ever source of potassium, which is why they're the one exception to the only-5-grams-at-a-time carb rule. Enjoy them often!

Just make your omelet according to Dana's Easy Omelet Method (page 57). Add the cheese, turn the burner to low, cover, and let the cheese melt. Add the avocado just before folding.

1½ teaspoons bacon grease

2 eggs, beaten

3 tablespoons (24 g) crumbled blue cheese

1 tablespoon (14 g) butter

1 tablespoon (15 ml) hot sauce (preferably Frank's RedHot, or Tabasco or Louisiana brand)

YIELD: 1 serving

384 calories: 34 g fat; 17 g protein; 2 g carbohydrate; 0 g dietary fiber per serving

BUFFALO WING OMELET

I had leftover buffalo wing sauce and thought of this. It turned out great! You could use bottled buffalo wing sauce if you have some on hand, but half-and-half, melted butter, and Frank's RedHot is the canonical recipe.

Make your omelet according to Dana's Easy Omelet Method (page 57) using the bacon grease for the fat. Fill with the blue cheese.

While your omelet is covered on low heat, melting the cheese, melt the butter with the Tabasco sauce in a small saucepan or nuke for a minute in a custard cup. Stir them together well.

When your omelet's done, fold and plate, and then top with the sauce and eat. Yummy!

1 tablespoon (15 ml) olive oil

2 eggs, beaten

2 tablespoons (20 g) crumbled feta cheese

2 tablespoons (14 g) shredded kasseri cheese

½ cup (28 g) chopped fresh spinach or baby spinach leaves

4 kalamata olives, pitted and chopped

YIELD: 1 serving

457 calories; 40 g fat; 21 g protein; 4 g carbohydrate; trace dietary fiber per serving

GREEK CHEESE, SPINACH, AND OLIVE OMELET

If you can't find kasseri, you can just double the feta. Or you can substitute shredded Romano; I find the flavor similar.

Make your omelet according to Dana's Easy Omelet Method (page 57), using the olive oil for the fat. Layer in the cheeses, then the spinach, with the chopped olives on top. Let it cook till the cheese is hot and the spinach just starting to wilt a bit.

---

2 slices bacon

2 ounces (55 g) sliced turkey breast

½ small tomato

1 scallion

2 eggs

1 tablespoon (14 g) mayonnaise

YIELD: 1 serving

383 calories; 28 g fat; 29 g protein; 5 g carbohydrate; 1 g dietary fiber per serving

CLUB OMELET

One of the few high-carb meals I miss is the turkey club sandwich, so here's the omelet equivalent. I developed this using deli turkey, but what a great breakfast for the weekend after Thanksgiving!

Cook and drain your bacon—I like to microwave mine and crumble it up. Cut the turkey into small squares, and slice the tomato and scallion.

Beat the eggs, and make your omelet according to Dana's Easy Omelet Method (page 57), using a couple of spoonfuls of the bacon grease. Add just the bacon and turkey before covering. Once it's cooked to your liking, sprinkle the tomato and scallion over the meat, spread the mayonnaise on the other side, fold, and serve.

1 tablespoon (15 ml) olive oil

2 eggs, beaten

2 ounces (55 g) Monterey Jack cheese, shredded

¼ avocado, sliced

¼ cup (4 g) alfalfa sprouts

YIELD: 1 serving

545 calories; 47 g fat; 26 g protein; 5 g carbohydrate; 1 g dietary fiber per serving

CALIFORNIA OMELET

I've had breakfast down near the waterfront in San Diego. This is what it tastes like. Beachfront ambience is up to you.

Make your omelet according to Dana's Easy Omelet Method (page 57), placing the Monterey Jack over half of your omelet when you're ready to add the filling. Cover, turn the heat to low, and cook until the cheese is melted (2 to 3 minutes). Arrange the avocado and sprouts over the cheese, and follow the directions to finish making the omelet.

1 tablespoon (14 g) butter

2 eggs, beaten

2 ounces (55 g) braunschweiger (liverwurst), mashed a bit with a fork

¼ medium ripe tomato, sliced

Mayonnaise (optional)

YIELD: 1 serving

443 calories; 39 g fat; 19 g protein; 4 g carbohydrate; trace dietary fiber per serving

BRAUNSCHWEIGER OMELET

Hey, don't make that face! Some of us love liverwurst! And this is an easy way to get the extraordinary nutrition of liver into your diet. Read the labels, by the way—my grocery store carries two brands of braunschweiger, one with just 1 gram of carb per serving, and one with 4 grams. Yeesh.

Make your omelet according to Dana's Easy Omelet Method (page 57), spooning the mashed braunschweiger over half of your omelet and topping with the tomato slices. If you'd like to gild the lily, a dollop of mayonnaise is good on top of this.

2 canned artichoke hearts

2 scallions

1 ounce (28 g) Monterey Jack cheese

3 eggs

1 teaspoon pesto sauce

1 tablespoon (14 g) butter

YIELD: 2 servings

449 calories; 36 g fat; 26 g protein; 5 g carbohydrate; trace dietary fiber per serving

MONTEREY SCRAMBLE

Named for the cheese, not the town, though this has a sort of California feel to me. This would make a nice quick supper.

Thinly slice your artichoke hearts, slice your scallions, shred your cheese and have them standing by. Scramble up your eggs with the pesto until it is completely blended in.

Give your medium skillet a squirt of nonstick cooking spray, and put it over medium-high heat. Add the butter and let it melt.

Throw your veggies in the skillet, and pour the eggs in on top of them. Scramble it all together, until the eggs are set almost to your liking. Scatter the cheese over the top, cover the skillet, turn off the burner, and let the residual heat melt the cheese and finish cooking the eggs.

4 eggs

½ cup (120 ml) heavy cream

1 teaspoon dried dill weed

4 scallions

4 ounces (115 g) chèvre (goat cheese)

4 ounces (115 g) moist smoked salmon

1 to 2 tablespoons (14 to 28 g) butter

YIELD: 3 servings

407 calories; 31 g fat; 27 g protein; 5 g carbohydrate; 1 g dietary fiber per serving

SMOKED SALMON AND GOAT CHEESE SCRAMBLE

Sounds fancy, I know, but this takes almost no time and is very impressive. It's terrific to make for a special brunch or a late-night supper. A simple green salad with a classic vinaigrette dressing would be perfect with this.

Whisk the eggs together with the cream and dill. Slice the scallions thin, including the crisp part of the green. Cut the chèvre—it will have a texture similar to cream cheese—into little hunks. Coarsely crumble the smoked salmon.

In a large (preferably nonstick) skillet, melt the butter over medium-high heat. (If your skillet doesn't have a nonstick surface, give it a shot of nonstick cooking spray before adding the butter.) When the butter's melted, add the scallions first, and sauté them for just a minute. Add the egg mixture and cook, stirring frequently, until the eggs are halfway set—about 60 to 90 seconds. Add the chèvre and smoked salmon, continue cooking and stirring until the eggs are set, and serve.

6 eggs

½ cup (50 g) grated Parmesan cheese

¼ cup (60 ml) heavy cream

1 teaspoon ground rosemary

1 clove garlic, crushed

1 tablespoon (14 g) butter

YIELD: 2 servings

448 calories; 36 g fat; 26 g protein; 4 g carbohydrate; trace dietary fiber per serving

4 ounces (115 g) bulk pork sausage

¼ cup (38 g) diced green bell pepper

¼ cup (38 g) diced red bell pepper

¼ cup (40 g) diced sweet red onion

¼ cup (25 g) grated Parmesan cheese

1 teaspoon original flavor Mrs. Dash

8 eggs, beaten

YIELD: 4 servings

279 calories; 22 g fat; 16 g protein; 4 g carbohydrate; 1 g dietary fiber per serving

PARMESAN-ROSEMARY EGGS

This is so simple and so wonderful. If you like Italian food, you have to try this. It's also easy to double or triple. You can use whole, dried rosemary, but you'll have little needles in your food. If you do use whole rosemary, increase the amount to 2 teaspoons.

Whisk together the eggs, cheese, cream, rosemary, and garlic. Put a large skillet over medium-high heat (if it isn't nonstick, give it a shot of nonstick cooking spray first). When the pan is hot, add the butter, give the egg mixture one last stir to make sure the cheese hasn't settled to the bottom, then pour the egg mixture into the skillet. Scramble until the eggs are set, and serve.

CONFETTI FRITTATA

The frittata is the Italian version of the omelet, and it involves no folding! If you're still intimidated by omelets, try a frittata. This is a good family supper. It's also good for making ahead, so you can just microwave a slice in the morning.

Preheat the broiler.

In a large, ovenproof skillet, start browning and crumbling the sausage over medium heat. As some fat starts to cook out of it, add the peppers and onion to the skillet. Cook the sausage and veggies until there's no pink left in the sausage. Spread the sausage-and-veggie mixture into an even layer in the bottom of the skillet.

In a medium bowl, beat the Parmesan cheese and seasoning into the eggs and pour the mixture over the sausage and veggies in the skillet.

Turn the heat to low and cover the skillet. (If your skillet doesn't have a cover, use foil.) Let the frittata cook until the eggs are mostly set. This may take up to 25 or 30 minutes, but the size of your skillet will affect the speed of cooking, so check periodically.

When all but the very top of the frittata is set, slide it under the broiler for about 5 minutes, or until the top is golden. Cut into wedges, and serve.

8 slices bacon

5 eggs

¼ cup (60 ml) heavy cream

¼ cup (60 ml) carb-reduced milk or sugar-free almond milk

1 tablespoon (15 ml) dry vermouth

½ teaspoon salt

¼ teaspoon ground black pepper

1 pinch ground nutmeg

1 tablespoon (14 g) butter

8 ounces (225 g) shredded Swiss cheese

YIELD: 4 servings

438 calories: 34 g fat; 28 g protein; 4 g carbohydrate; trace dietary fiber per serving

INSTA-QUICHE

As the name implies, this has a similar flavor to a classic quiche lorraine, but it cooks in 15 minutes' time. Doesn't need a crust, either.

Place a 10-inch (25 cm) nonstick skillet over medium heat. Let it heat.

Lay the bacon on a microwave bacon rack or in a microwavable baking dish. Stick it in the microwave on high for 8 to 9 minutes. (The length of time will depend a bit on your microwave.)

In a medium mixing bowl, whisk together the eggs, cream, carb-reduced milk, vermouth, salt, pepper, and nutmeg.

Put your butter in your now-hot skillet and swirl it around as it melts to coat the bottom. Now pour in your egg mixture. Use a spatula—preferably one for nonstick skillets—to gently stir the eggs around, pulling back the part that's setting and letting the liquid egg run underneath. It won't work like an omelet, where it sets up firm enough that you can lift the whole edge. Just scramble them gently until they're about half-set, half-liquid.

Spread the eggs out evenly in the skillet and sprinkle the shredded cheese over the top. Cover the skillet and turn the burner to low. (If you have an electric stove, you'll need to shift your pan to a low burner.) Turn on the broiler and set the rack 4 inches (10 cm) below it.

When the bacon is done, take it out, drain it, and let it cool just a minute or two. Then crumble it, or easier, you can use your kitchen shears to snip it into bits. Uncover your Insta-Quiche and sprinkle the bacon bits evenly over the top.

Now slide the whole thing under the broiler for just a minute until you're sure the top is set, then cut into wedges and serve.

¼ head cauliflower

1 medium turnip

1 medium onion, sliced thin

2 to 3 tablespoons (30 to 45 ml) olive oil, divided

6 eggs

Salt and ground black pepper, to taste

Chopped fresh parsley (optional)

YIELD: 6 servings

139 calories; 11 g fat; 6 g protein; 4 g carbohydrate; 1 g dietary fiber per serving

UNPOTATO TORTILLA

Don't think Mexican flatbread, think eggs. In Spain, a tortilla is much like an Italian frittata—a substantial egg dish, cooked in a skillet and served in wedges. This one is my version of a traditional dish served in tapas bars all over Spain. As bar food goes, it's a heckuva step up from beer nuts and stale popcorn. This would make a great supper, or prepare it ahead and nuke a slice for a quick breakfast.

Prehead your broiler on low.

Thinly slice your cauliflower—include the stem—and peel and thinly slice your turnip. Put them in a microwaveable casserole dish with a lid, add a couple of tablespoons of water (about 40 ml), and microwave on high for 6 to 7 minutes.

In the meanwhile, start the onion sautéing in 2 tablespoons (30 ml) of the olive oil in an 8- to 9-inch (20 to 23 cm) skillet—a nonstick skillet is ideal, but not essential. If your skillet isn't nonstick, give it a good squirt of nonstick cooking spray first. Use medium heat.

When your microwave goes beep, pull out the veggies, drain them, and throw them in the skillet with the onion. Continue sautéing everything, adding a bit more oil if things start to stick, until the veggies are getting golden around the edges—about 10 to 15 minutes. Turn the heat to low and spread the vegetables in an even layer on the bottom of the skillet.

Mix up the eggs with a little salt and pepper and pour over the vegetables. Cook on low for 5 to 7 minutes, lifting the edges frequently to let uncooked egg run underneath. When it's all set except for the top, slide the skillet under a low broiler for 4 to 5 minutes, or until the top of your tortilla is golden. (If your skillet doesn't have a flameproof handle, wrap it in foil first.) Cut into wedges to serve. A little chopped parsley is nice on this, but not essential.

1 pound (455 g) asparagus

1 clove garlic, crushed

¼ cup (60 ml) olive oil

Salt and ground black pepper, to taste

½ cup (50 g) grated Parmesan cheese

8 eggs

YIELD: 4 servings

310 calories; 25 g fat; 16 g protein; 4 g carbohydrate; 1 g dietary fiber per serving

ASPARAGI ALL'UOVO

This Italian dish turns a couple of eggs into a light supper. This looks like a lot of instructions, but none of the steps takes much time.

Preheat the broiler.

Snap the bottoms off the asparagus where they break naturally. Put the asparagus spears in a microwavable casserole dish or a glass pie plate. Add a couple of tablespoons of water (40 ml) and cover. (Use plastic wrap or a plate to cover a pie plate.) Microwave on high for 3 to 4 minutes.

While the asparagus is cooking, crush the garlic into the olive oil.

When the asparagus is done, drain it. If you have 4 gratin dishes—long, oval single-serving ovenproof dishes—they're ideal for this recipe. Divide the asparagus among the 4 dishes. If not, you'll need to use a rectangular glass baking dish. Arrange the asparagus in 4 groups in the baking dish.

Whether you're using the individual dishes or the single baking dish, drizzle each serving of asparagus with the garlic oil. Sprinkle lightly with salt and pepper and divide the cheese among the 4 servings. Put the asparagus under the broiler, about 4 inches (10 cm) from low heat. Let it broil for 4 to 5 minutes.

While the asparagus is broiling, fry the eggs to your liking. Either use your biggest skillet to do them all at once, or divide them between 2 skillets.

When the Parmesan is lightly golden, take the asparagus out of the broiler. If you've cooked it in one baking dish, use a big spatula to carefully transfer each serving of asparagus to a plate. Top each serving of asparagus with 2 fried eggs, and serve.

4 slices bacon, chopped into 1-inch (2.5 cm) pieces

4 thin slices onion—round slices through the equator

4 eggs

4 thin slices Cheddar cheese—1-ounce (28 g) square deli slices (or a few thin slices off the end of an 8-ounce (225 g) block)

YIELD: 2 servings

438 calories; 34 g fat; 29 g protein; 3 g carbohydrate; trace dietary fiber per serving

1 clove garlic

3 tablespoons (45 ml) olive oil

⅓ cup (80 g) no-sugar-added pizza sauce*

1½ teaspoon dried oregano

½ teaspoon red pepper flakes (optional)

¼ cup (25 g) grated Parmesan cheese

YIELD: 6 servings

262 calories; 22 g fat; 14 g protein; 3 g carbohydrate; trace dietary fiber per serving

*To find no-sugar-added pizza sauce, read labels. My favorite is made by Pastorelli, a Chicagoland brand, that I can now get here in southern Indiana. Ragu makes one—it's labeled just "Pizza Sauce," not "Pizza Quick Sauce." Muir Glen, a brand available in health food stores and some supermarkets, has one, too.

RODEO EGGS

This was originally a sandwich recipe, but it works just as well without the bread.

Begin frying the bacon in a heavy skillet over medium heat. When some fat has cooked out of it, push it aside and put the onion slices in, too. Fry the onion on each side, turning carefully to keep the slices together, until it starts to look translucent. Remove the onion from the skillet and set aside.

Continue frying the bacon until it's crisp. Pour off most of the grease and distribute the bacon bits evenly over the bottom of the skillet. Break in the eggs and fry for a minute or two, until the bottoms are set but the tops are still soft. (If you like your yolks hard, break them with a fork; if you like them soft, leave them unbroken.)

Place a slice of onion over each yolk, then cover the onion with a slice of cheese. Add a teaspoon of water to the skillet, cover, and cook for 2 to 3 minutes, or until the cheese is thoroughly melted.

Cut into 4 separate pieces with the edge of a spatula, and serve.

BACKWARDS PIZZA

With America's love for pizza, it's not surprising that low-carb pizza crust recipes abound. I decided to try just cheese. It worked out remarkably well. Once it cools a bit, you can eat this with your hands, like regular pizza.

Preheat oven to 375°F (190°C, or gas mark 5). Line a jelly roll tin with nonstick foil (Reynolds makes this).

Spread the mozzarella evenly over the foil, all the way to the corners. Bake for 5 minutes, turn the pan to help it cook evenly, and give it another 5 to 7 minutes—you want the cheese golden brown all over.

While the cheese is baking, crush the garlic into a little cup and cover with the olive oil, stirring once.

Put your pizza sauce in a microwavable dish, and give it 1 minute to warm.

When your cheese is an even, golden layer, pull it out of the oven. Drizzle the garlicky oil all over it, spreading with a brush or the back of a spoon. Sprinkle with oregano and red pepper flakes if using.

Spread the pizza sauce over the oil, and sprinkle the Parmesan over that.

Cut into 6 big rectangles to serve.

CHAPTER 6
Side Salads

Since everything leafy falls into the "very low carb" category, salads are a good bet. Your grocery store should have a wide variety of bagged salad, ready to dress and eat. But you must watch out for dressings. First of all, skip all "lite," low-fat, or fat-free dressings. Chances are high that they've replaced the fat with corn syrup or some other kind of sugar. You also need to watch out for any dressing that actually tastes sweet—poppy seed, Catalina and that red "French" stuff, honey mustard, raspberry vinaigrette, all of those. Need I warn you again? Read the labels.

Bottled full-fat dressings that are generally safe include ranch, blue cheese, and Caesar.

Some vinaigrettes—my favorite kind of dressing—are okay, but be careful. Balsamic vinaigrette and raspberry vinaigrette, in particular, may be carb heavy. There's a raspberry vinaigrette dressing here!

In this chapter, you'll also find a wide variety of deli-style salads, the sort of thing you can make when you have time, stash in the fridge, and pull out at the last minute. These are a great alternative to the potato or macaroni salad and sugary coleslaw sold at the grocery store deli. The busier you are, the handier this kind of thing will be.

The dressing recipes are at the end of this chapter. First, let's go for some salads.

6 cups (330 g) torn romaine lettuce hearts

3 tablespoons (45 ml) extra-virgin olive oil

1½ tablespoons (23 g) pesto sauce

⅓ cup (40 g) crumbled Gorgonzola cheese

YIELD: 4 servings
163 calories; 16 g fat; 4 g protein; 3 g carbohydrate; 2 g dietary fiber per serving

GORGONZOLA-AND-PESTO CAESAR SALAD

Oh, all right, use another blue cheese if you must. But being Italian and all, Gorgonzola is best here.

This is super-simple! Put your lettuce in a big salad bowl. Mix the olive oil and pesto together and then pour over the salad and toss furiously until it's all evenly coated. Sprinkle the Gorgonzola over the whole thing, toss lightly again, and serve.

4 cups (120 g) fresh spinach

⅛ large sweet red onion, thinly sliced

3 tablespoons (45 ml) oil—light olive oil or MCT oil

2 tablespoons (28 ml) cider vinegar

2 teaspoons tomato paste

9 drops liquid stevia (plain)

¼ small onion, grated

⅛ teaspoon dry mustard

Salt and ground black pepper, to taste

2 slices bacon, cooked until crisp, and crumbled

1 hard-boiled egg, chopped

YIELD: 3 servings
315 calories; 29 g fat; 11 g protein; 4 g carbohydrate; 1 g dietary fiber per serving

CLASSIC SPINACH SALAD

A mid-twentieth-century classic, spinach salad with a slightly sweet dressing, topped with bacon and hard-boiled egg, never grows old.

Wash the spinach very well and dry. Tear up larger leaves. Combine with the onion in a salad bowl.

In a separate bowl, mix up the oil, vinegar, tomato paste, Stevia, grated red onion, mustard, and salt and pepper to taste. Pour the mixture over the spinach and onion, and toss.

Top each serving with bacon and egg.

2 cucumbers, scrubbed but not peeled

1 green bell pepper

½ large sweet red onion

½ head cauliflower

2 teaspoons salt or Vege-Sal

1 cup (230 g) sour cream

2 tablespoons (28 ml) vinegar (cider vinegar is best, but wine vinegar will do)

2 rounded teaspoons dried dill weed

YIELD: 10 servings

64 calories; 5 g fat; 1 g protein; 4 g carbohydrate; 1 g dietary fiber per serving

½ head cauliflower

⅔ cup (70 g) sliced stuffed olives (you can buy 'em pre-sliced in jars)

7 scallions, sliced

2 cups (60 g) triple-washed fresh spinach, finely chopped

1 rib celery, diced

1 small ripe tomato, finely diced

¼ cup (15 g) chopped fresh parsley

¼ cup (60 ml) olive oil

2 tablespoons (28 g) mayonnaise

1 tablespoon (15 ml) red wine vinegar

1 teaspoon minced garlic or 2 cloves garlic, crushed

Salt and ground black pepper, to taste

YIELD: 6 servings

148 calories; 15 g fat; 1 g protein; 5 g carbohydrate; 2 g dietary fiber per serving

SOUR CREAM AND CUKE SALAD

Très 1950s—and so good! Better, it improves with a day in the refrigerator, so it's a great make-ahead dish.

Slice the cucumbers, pepper, onion, and cauliflower as thinly as you possibly can. The slicing blade on a food processor works nicely, and it saves you mucho time, but I've also done it with a good, sharp knife.

Toss the vegetables well with the salt, and chill them in the refrigerator for an hour or two.

In a separate bowl, mix the sour cream, vinegar, and dill, combining well.

Remove the veggies from the fridge, drain off any water that has collected at the bottom of the bowl, and stir in the sour cream mixture. Refrigerate for at least a few hours before serving.

NOT-QUITE-MIDDLE-EASTERN SALAD

Here shredded cauliflower "rice" stands in for bulgur wheat. This salad is incredibly delicious, incredibly nutritious, and quite beautiful on the plate. Plus, it gets better after a couple of days in the fridge, so taking an extra few minutes to double the batch is definitely worth it. For a main-dish salad, add diced cooked chicken, lump crabmeat, or shrimp.

Prepare the cauliflower as for Cauli-Rice, page 78. Give it just 6 minutes of microwave steaming.

While that's cooking, prep the olives, scallions, spinach, celery, tomato, and parsley and combine in a large salad bowl.

When the cauliflower comes out of the microwave, dump it into a strainer and run cold water over it for a moment or two to cool it. (You can let the cauliflower cool, uncovered, instead, but it will take longer.) Drain the cauliflower well and dump it in with all the other vegetables. Add the oil, mayonnaise, vinegar, and garlic, and toss. Add salt and pepper to taste, toss again, and serve.

1 large head cauliflower, cut into small chunks

2 cups (240 g) diced celery

1 cup (160 g) diced red onion

2 cups (450 g) mayonnaise

¼ cup (60 ml) cider vinegar

2 teaspoons salt or Vege-Sal

½ teaspoon ground black pepper

12 drops liquid stevia (plain)

4 hard-boiled eggs, chopped

YIELD: 12 servings

298 calories; 33 g fat; 3 g protein; 2 g carbohydrate; 1 g dietary fiber per serving

UNPOTATO SALAD

You are going to be so surprised; this is amazingly like potato salad. I have seen people take two or three bites before they figure out it's not potatoes. This is modeled on the old-school picnic favorite.

Put the cauliflower in a microwavable casserole dish, add just a tablespoon (15 ml) or so of water, and cover. Cook it on high for 7 minutes, and let it sit, covered, for another 3 to 5 minutes. You want your cauliflower tender, but not mushy. (And you may steam it on the stove top, if you prefer.)

Use the time while the cauliflower cooks to dice your celery and onion.

Drain the cooked cauliflower and combine it with the celery and onion in a really big bowl.

In a separate bowl, combine the mayonnaise, vinegar, salt, pepper, and stevia. Pour the mixture over the vegetables and mix well. Mix in the chopped eggs last, and only stir lightly, to preserve some small hunks of yolk. Chill and serve.

½ head cauliflower

½ cup (115 g) mayonnaise

2 tablespoons (22 g) spicy mustard

1 tablespoon (15 ml) lime juice

1 small jalapeño

⅓ cup (5 g) chopped fresh cilantro

⅓ cup (55 g) diced red onion

1 clove garlic, crushed

1 small tomato

YIELD: 6 servings

158 calories; 16 g fat; 2 g protein; 5 g carbohydrate; 2 g dietary fiber per serving

SOUTHWESTERN UNPOTATO SALAD

I have tried at least a couple dozen potato salad recipes using cauliflower instead, and not a one has failed. But of all the "unpotato" salads I've come up with, this one is my favorite!

First, cut your cauliflower into ½-inch (1 cm) chunks—don't bother coring it first, just trim the bottom of the stem and cut up the core with the rest of it. Put your cauliflower chunks in a microwavable casserole dish with a lid, add a few tablespoons of water (about 40 ml), and cook it on high for 7 minutes.

When your cauliflower is done, drain it and put it in a large mixing bowl. In a medium bowl, whisk together the mayonnaise, mustard, and lime juice; then pour it over the cauliflower and mix well.

Cut the jalapeño in half, remove the seeds, and mince it fine. Add it to the salad along with the cilantro, onion, and garlic; mix again (don't forget to wash your hands!).

Finally, cut the stem out of the tomato and cut the tomato into smallish dice, then carefully stir it in. Chill the salad for a few hours before serving.

½ head cauliflower

8 ounces (225 g) bacon, cooked until crisp, and crumbled

1 large tomato, chopped

10 scallions, sliced, including all the crisp part of the green

½ cup (115 g) mayonnaise

Salt and ground black pepper, to taste

Lettuce (optional)

YIELD: 6 servings

374 calories; 34 g fat; 13 g protein; 5 g carbohydrate; 2 g dietary fiber per serving

BACON, TOMATO, AND CAULIFLOWER SALAD

This recipe originally called for cooked rice, so I thought I'd try it with cauliflower "rice." I liked it so much, I ate it all and made it again the very next day.

Put the cauliflower through a food processor with the shredding disk. Steam or microwave it until it's tender-crisp (about 5 minutes on high in a microwave).

Combine the cooked cauliflower with the bacon, tomato, scallions, and mayonnaise in a big bowl. Add salt and pepper to taste and mix.

This salad holds a molded shape really well, so you can pack it into a custard cup and unmold it onto a plate lined with lettuce, if desired; it looks quite pretty served this way.

---

1 pound (455 g) asparagus

4 teaspoons (20 ml) soy sauce

2 teaspoons dark sesame oil

1 tablespoon (8 g) sesame seeds

YIELD: 4 servings

50 calories; 4 g fat; 2 g protein; 4 g carbohydrate; 2 g dietary fiber per serving

SESAME-ASPARAGUS SALAD

This unusual salad is a great way to celebrate the spring abundance of asparagus. Easy, too!

Snap the ends off your asparagus where they want to break naturally. Cut the spears into 1½-inch (3.5 cm) lengths, and put them in a microwave steamer or a microwavable casserole dish with a lid. Either way, add a couple of tablespoons of water (40 ml), cover, and microwave for just 3 to 4 minutes —you want it brilliantly green and just barely tender-crisp. Undercooking is better than overcooking!

Uncover your asparagus as soon as the microwave beeps to stop the cooking. Drain well, and put in a deep, narrow bowl.

Combine the soy sauce and sesame oil. Pour over the asparagus, and toss. Chill for an hour or two.

When ready to serve, put the sesame seeds in a small, dry skillet over medium-low heat, and shake them until they start to "pop"—jump a bit— and smell toasty. Remove from the heat. Stir the sesame seeds into the asparagus, and serve immediately.

¾ cup (180 ml) extra-virgin olive oil

⅓ cup (80 ml) wine vinegar

1 teaspoon Dijon mustard

1 clove garlic, crushed

½ teaspoon salt

¼ teaspoon ground black pepper

YIELD: 12 servings or 9 fluid ounces (265 ml)—a little more than a cup

121 calories; 14 g fat; trace protein; 1 g carbohydrate; trace dietary fiber per serving

⅔ cup (160 ml) extra-virgin olive oil

⅓ cup (80 ml) wine vinegar

½ teaspoon salt

½ teaspoon dried oregano

¼ teaspoon dried basil

¼ teaspoon ground black pepper

1 tiny pinch red pepper flakes

2 cloves garlic, crushed

YIELD: 12 servings or 1 cup (235 ml)

108 calories; 12 g fat; trace protein; 1 g carbohydrate; trace dietary fiber per serving

FRENCH VINAIGRETTE

No, this is not that sweet, tomatoey goo that somehow has gotten the name "French dressing." No Frenchman would eat that stuff on a bet! This is a classic oil-and-vinegar dressing.

Just put everything in a clean jar, lid it tightly, and shake vigorously. You can store it in the jar and just shake it up again before use.

ITALIAN VINAIGRETTE

Add a little zip to the French Vinaigrette, and you've got Italian Vinaigrette.

Assemble everything in a jar, lid it tightly, and shake-shake-shake. Store it in the jar in the fridge, and just shake it again before using.

VARIATION: Creamy Italian Dressing

Just add 2 tablespoons (28 g) of mayonnaise to the Italian Vinaigrette and whisk or shake until smooth.

½ cup (120 ml) light olive oil

¼ cup (60 ml) cider vinegar

¼ cup (45 g) brown mustard

⅛ teaspoon liquid stevia (plain)

¼ teaspoon ground black pepper

¼ teaspoon salt

YIELD: 12 servings or a generous 1 cup (235 ml)

6 calories; trace fat; trace protein; 1 g carbohydrate; trace dietary fiber per serving

TANGY "HONEY" MUSTARD DRESSING

You know that despite being "natural," honey is pure sugar, right? Make this instead. For a creamy version, substitute mayonnaise for half of the olive oil.

Just assemble everything in a clean jar, lid it tightly, and shake like mad. Store in the fridge, right in the jar, and shake again before using.

½ cup (115 g) mayonnaise

½ cup (115 g) sour cream

1 to 1½ tablespoons (15 to 23 ml) cider vinegar

1 to 1½ teaspoons prepared mustard

½ to 1 teaspoon salt or Vege-Sal

12 drops liquid stevia (plain)

YIELD: 8 servings or a generous 1 cup (235 ml)

132 calories; 15 g fat; 1 g protein; 1 g carbohydrate; trace dietary fiber per serving

COLESLAW DRESSING

Virtually all commercial coleslaw dressing is simply full of sugar, which is a shame, because cabbage is a very low-carb vegetable. I just love coleslaw, so I came up with a sugar-free dressing. You may, of course, vary these proportions to taste. Also, a teaspoon or so of celery seed can be nice in this for a little variety. I use this much dressing for a whole head of cabbage, shredded. Or take the easy route and use bagged coleslaw mix.

Combine all the ingredients well and toss with coleslaw mix.

½ shallot

½ teaspoon Dijon mustard

¼ cup (60 ml) raspberry vinegar—read the labels to find one with no sugar

6 drops liquid stevia (plain)

½ cup (120 ml) olive oil

Salt and ground black pepper, to taste

YIELD: 8 servings or ¾ cup (175 ml)

121 calories; 14 g fat; trace protein; 1 g carbohydrate; trace dietary fiber per serving

---

RASPBERRY VINAIGRETTE

Raspberry vinegar varies; some brands have sugar, and some do not, so be vigilant in reading labels. This is great on any salad that has a salty ingredient—feta, bacon, that sort of thing.

Put the shallot and mustard in your food processor, and turn it on. As the shallots are reaching the minced stage, add the raspberry vinegar and liquid stevia. Now slowly pour in the olive oil. When it's well incorporated, turn off the processor.

Taste, add salt and pepper, then pulse just another second or two to mix, and it's ready to use.

---

4 cups (280 g) finely shredded napa cabbage

¼ cup (30 g) shredded carrot

¼ cup (30 g) thinly sliced celery—the pale, inner part of the rib bunch

2 scallions, thinly sliced

¼ cup (60 g) mayonnaise

2 tablespoons (28 ml) rice vinegar

1 teaspoon grated fresh ginger root

1 teaspoon soy sauce

6 drops liquid stevia (plain)

YIELD: 8 servings

63 calories; 6 g fat; 1 g protein; 3 g carbohydrate; 1 g dietary fiber per serving

---

ASIAN GINGER SLAW

Even my slaw-hating husband likes this! It's got a very different texture and flavor than your standard slaw.

Combine the cabbage, carrot, celery, and scallions in a salad bowl.

In a separate bowl, combine the mayonnaise, vinegar, ginger, soy sauce, and stevia. Beat together until smooth, pour over the vegetables, toss, and serve.

12 cups (360 g) baby spinach

2 red plums

2 scallions, sliced

2 tablespoons (28 ml) peanut oil, light olive oil, or MCT oil

2 tablespoons (28 ml) rice vinegar

1 teaspoon soy sauce

½ teaspoon grated fresh ginger root

3 drops liquid stevia (plain)

YIELD: 8 servings

51 calories; 4 g fat; 2 g protein; 4 g carbohydrate; 2 g dietary fiber per serving

(NS) SPINACH-PLUM SALAD

The light Asian-style dressing with the sweet plums is quite extraordinary. This would be nice with a simple chicken dish, or perhaps white fish of some kind.

Dump your baby spinach in your big salad bowl.

Halve the plums, remove the pits, and cut into ½-inch (1 cm) dice. Slice your scallions, including the crisp part of the green.

In a small bowl, whisk together the peanut oil, rice vinegar, soy sauce, ginger, and stevia. Pour this over the spinach and toss till it's coated with the dressing. Pile the spinach on 8 salad plates, top each serving with plum cubes and scallions, and serve.

4 cups (220 g) torn romaine lettuce

4 cups (220 g) torn leaf lettuce

2 cups (110 g) torn arugula

2 cups (110 g) torn radicchio

2 ounces (55 g) goat cheese

3 tablespoons (23 g) chopped walnuts

½ cup (120 ml) Raspberry Vinaigrette (page 74)

¼ cup (30 g) fresh raspberries

YIELD: 5 servings

229 calories; 21 g fat; 6 g protein; 5 g carbohydrate; 2 g dietary fiber per serving

(NS) MIXED GREENS WITH WALNUTS, GOAT CHEESE, AND RASPBERRY DRESSING

The slightly bitter greens, the sweet dressing, the creamy goat cheese, and the crispy nuts make a heckuva combination!

Assemble your lettuces, arugula, and radicchio in your salad bowl. Cut your goat cheese into little hunks. Chop your walnuts and have 'em standing by.

Now pour your dressing over the greens, and toss. Pile the salad onto 5 salad plates, and top each with a little goat cheese, some walnuts, and a few raspberries.

1 clove garlic

½ cup (120 ml) extra-virgin olive oil

1 head romaine lettuce

½ cup (30 g) chopped fresh parsley

½ green bell pepper, diced

¼ cucumber, quartered and sliced

¼ sweet red onion, sliced paper-thin

2 to 3 tablespoons (30 to 45 ml) lemon juice

2 to 3 teaspoons (10 to 15 ml) Worcestershire sauce

¼ cup (25 g) grated Parmesan cheese

1 medium ripe tomato, cut into thin wedges

YIELD: 8 servings
156 calories; 14 g fat; 3 g protein; 5 g carbohydrate; 2 g dietary fiber per serving

DANA AND ERIC'S FAVORITE SALAD

If you're looking for a standard tossed salad, this is as good as it gets. The combination of flavors is stunning. My husband and I have served this salad over and over, and we never tire of it. This dressing tastes a bit like a Caesar vinaigrette, but it's less trouble.

Crush the clove of garlic in a small bowl, cover it with the olive oil, and set it aside.

Wash and dry your romaine, break it up into a bowl, and add the parsley, pepper, cucumber, and onion. Pour the garlic-flavored oil over the salad and toss until every leaf is covered.

Sprinkle on the lemon juice to taste and toss again. Then sprinkle on the Worcestershire sauce as desired and toss again. Finally, sprinkle on the Parmesan and toss one last time. Top with the tomato wedges, and serve.

CHAPTER 7
Hot Vegetable Dishes

You're used to diets that tell you to eat tons of vegetables, aren't you? And to leave off the butter, oil, and sour cream, because they're—*gasp*—fat.

Prepare for a paradigm shift. If you have diabetes, or even prediabetes, you need to keep an eye on all carbs, even those from vegetables. Remember, a molecule of glucose is a molecule of glucose, regardless of the source.

Vegetables will be the source of most of your carbs. To stay at 20 grams or fewer per day, we're talking just a couple of cups of vegetables per day. Some of the higher carb vegetables have to be limited even more strictly, and the really starchy ones—peas, lima beans, corn, and the like—are out entirely.

You did not get sick from eating vegetables. But with a broken carbohydrate metabolism you have to watch all carbohydrates. The recipes here with 5 grams per serving can accompany plain protein courses—a grilled steak, a pan-broiled chop, roast chicken, and the like. As you heal, you may be able to increase vegetable portions—that will be between you, your glucometer, and your doctor.

All of that said, it's vegetables that are going to vary the meat, poultry, fish, and eggs that will be the core of your diet. I think you'll be surprised how much they—*ahem*—bring to the table. Feel free to serve your vegetables steamed with a little melted butter. Simple is good. But for those times when you want something a bit more interesting, here's a fine variety of pleasing vegetable dishes.

1 head cauliflower (you need about 1½ pounds, or 680 g, total, fresh or frozen)

2 ounces (55 g) cream cheese

¼ cup (55 g) butter

Salt and ground black pepper, to taste

YIELD: 6 servings (or more)
125 calories; 11 g fat; 3 g protein; 5 g carbohydrate; 2 g dietary fiber per serving

½ head cauliflower

YIELD: 4 servings
18 calories; trace fat; 1 g protein; 4 g carbohydrate; 2 g dietary fiber per serving

CAULIFLOWER PURÉE (A.K.A. FAUXTATOES)

This is a wonderful substitute for mashed potatoes with any dish that has a gravy or sauce. Feel free to use frozen cauliflower; it works quite well here. You can steam your cauliflower on the stove top if you prefer.

Play with this! Stir in shredded cheese or a dollop of horseradish, or use chive cream cheese instead of plain.

Trim the very bottom of the cauliflower stem, and remove the leaves. Cut the rest into chunks. Put the cauliflower in a microwavable casserole dish with a lid, or a microwave steamer, add a couple of tablespoons (28 ml) of water, and cover. Microwave it on high for 12 minutes, or until quite tender but not sulfury smelling. Drain it thoroughly. Now puree it—I use my stick blender, but you can put it in your food processor if you prefer. Work in the cream cheese and butter, then season with salt and pepper to taste.

CAULI-RICE

With thanks to Fran McCullough! I got this idea from her book *Living Low-Carb*, and it's served me very well indeed. It makes a nice bed for a piece of chicken or fish with a tasty sauce, works as a base for great seasoned "rice" dishes, and even stands in for rice, couscous, or bulgur in salads.

Trim the leaves and the very bottom of the stem from your cauliflower. Cut it into chunks, and run them through the shredding blade of your food processor. Steam lightly—I add a little water and give mine 6 to 7 minutes on high in the microwave.

½ head cauliflower

2 eggs

1 cup (75 g) fresh snow pea pods

2 tablespoons (28 g) butter

½ cup (80 g) diced onion

2 tablespoons (16 g) shredded carrot

3 tablespoons (45 ml) soy sauce

Salt and ground black pepper, to taste

YIELD: 5 servings

91 calories; 6 g fat; 4 g protein; 5 g carbohydrate; 1 g dietary fiber per serving

JAPANESE FRIED "RICE"

A fine side dish, but it can be easily converted into a skillet supper with the addition of a protein. How about shrimp, or diced leftover rotisserie chicken or pork roast?

Turn your cauliflower into Cauli-Rice according to the instructions on page 78.

While that's happening, whisk the eggs, pour them into a nonstick skillet (or one you've coated with nonstick cooking spray), and cook over medium-high heat. As you cook the eggs, use your spatula to break them up into pea-sized bits. Remove from the skillet and set aside.

Remove the tips and strings from the snow peas and snip into ¼-inch (6 mm) lengths. (By now the microwave has beeped—take the lid off your cauliflower or it will turn into a mush that bears not the slightest resemblance to rice!)

Melt the butter in the skillet and sauté the pea pods, onion, and carrot for 2 to 3 minutes. Add the cauliflower and stir everything together well. Stir in the soy sauce and cook the whole thing, stirring often, for another 5 to 6 minutes. Add a little salt and pepper, and serve.

½ head cauliflower

½ medium onion, chopped

2 tablespoons (28 g) butter, divided

¼ cup (60 ml) dry white wine

1 tablespoon (18 g) chicken bouillon concentrate

1 teaspoon poultry seasoning

¼ cup (28 g) sliced or slivered almonds

YIELD: 5 servings

104 calories; 9 g fat; 2 g protein; 4 g carbohydrate; 1 g dietary fiber per serving

CHICKEN-ALMOND "RICE"

This is great for fans of rice pilaf mixes—my brother dubbed it "Rice-a-Phony." It's terrific with a simple rotisserie chicken.

Turn your cauliflower into Cauli-Rice according to the instructions on page 78.

While that's cooking, sauté the onion in 1 tablespoon (14 g) of the butter in a large, heavy skillet over medium-high heat.

When the cauliflower is done, pull it out of the microwave, drain it, and add it to the skillet with the onion. Add the wine, chicken bouillon concentrate, and poultry seasoning, and stir. Turn the heat down to low.

Let that simmer for a minute or two while you sauté the almonds in the remaining tablespoon (14 g) of butter in a small, heavy skillet. When the almonds are golden, stir them into the "rice," and serve.

½ head cauliflower

4 strips bacon

½ medium onion, chopped

2 tablespoons (30 g) tomato sauce

1 tablespoon (18 g) beef bouillon concentrate

2 tablespoons (18 g) toasted pine nuts

2 tablespoons (8 g) chopped fresh parsley

YIELD: 5 servings

72 calories; 4 g fat; 4 g protein; 5 g carbohydrate; 2 g dietary fiber per serving

½ head cauliflower

3 tablespoons (42 g) butter

1 cup (70 g) sliced mushrooms

½ medium onion, diced

1 teaspoon minced garlic or 2 cloves garlic, minced

2 tablespoons (28 ml) dry vermouth

1 tablespoon (18 g) chicken bouillon concentrate

¾ cup (75 g) grated Parmesan cheese

Guar or xanthan, as needed

2 tablespoons (8 g) chopped fresh parsley

YIELD: 5 servings

139 calories; 11 g fat; 6 g protein; 4 g carbohydrate; 1 g dietary fiber per serving

BEEF AND BACON "RICE" WITH PINE NUTS

A great side with a steak or burger. Or put this next to roast beef, and you've got a killer company dinner. Stir in slivered leftover roast beef, should you have any, and you have a skillet supper.

Turn your cauliflower into Cauli-Rice according to the instructions on page 78.

While that's cooking, cut the bacon into little pieces—kitchen shears are good for this—and start the little bacon bits frying in a heavy skillet over medium-high heat. When a little grease has cooked out of the bacon, throw the onion into the skillet. Cook until the onion is translucent and the bacon is browned and getting crisp.

By now the cauliflower should be done. Drain it and throw it in the skillet with the bacon and onion. Add the tomato sauce and beef bouillon concentrate, and stir the whole thing up to combine everything—you can add a couple of tablespoons (28 ml) of water, if you like, to help the liquid flavorings spread.

Stir in the pine nuts and parsley (you can just snip it right into the skillet with clean kitchen shears), and serve.

MUSHROOM "RISOTTO"

Man, is this good! One of the best side dishes I've ever come up with. I made this with Wayne Brady when I was on his talk show!

Turn your cauliflower into Cauli-Rice according to the instructions on page 78.

While the cauliflower is cooking, melt the butter in a large skillet over medium-high heat. Add the mushrooms, onion, and garlic, and sauté them all together.

When the cauliflower is done, pull it out of the microwave and drain it. When the mushrooms have changed color and are looking done, add the cauliflower to the skillet and stir everything together. Stir in the vermouth and bouillon, add the cheese, and let the whole thing cook for another 2 to 3 minutes.

Sprinkle just a little guar or xanthan over the "risotto," stirring all the while, to give it a creamy texture. Stir in the parsley just before serving.

4 slices bacon

½ head cauliflower

½ green bell pepper

½ medium onion

¼ cup (25 g) sliced stuffed olives

YIELD: 5 servings
49 calories; 4 g fat; 2 g protein;
3 g carbohydrate; 1 g dietary fiber
per serving

LITTLE MAMA'S SIDE DISH

This is just the thing with a simple dinner of broiled chops or a steak, and it's even good all by itself. It's beautiful to look at, too, what with all those colors, which is why I chose it to make on George Stella's Food Network show, *Low Carb and Lovin' It*. By the way, you can buy sliced stuffed olives in jars.

Chop the bacon into small bits and start it frying in a large, heavy skillet over medium-high heat. (Give the skillet a squirt of nonstick cooking spray first.)

Chop the cauliflower into ½-inch (1 cm) bits. Chop up the stem, too; no need to waste it. Put the chopped cauliflower in a microwavable casserole dish with a lid—or a microwave steamer if you have one—add a couple of tablespoons (28 ml) of water, cover, and microwave for 8 minutes on high.

Give the bacon a stir, then go back to the chopping board. Dice the pepper and onion. By now some fat has cooked out of the bacon, and it is starting to brown around the edges. Add the pepper and onion to the skillet. Sauté until the onion is translucent and the pepper is starting to get soft.

By then, the cauliflower should be done. Add it to the skillet without draining and stir—the extra little bit of water is going to help dissolve the yummy bacon flavor from the bottom of the skillet and carry it through the dish.

Stir in the olives, let the whole thing cook another minute while stirring, then serve.

1 head cauliflower, cut into florets (or 1½ pounds [680 g] frozen cauliflower)

1 large egg

1 cup (225 g) small-curd whole-milk cottage cheese

1 cup (230 g) sour cream

½ teaspoon salt

⅛ teaspoon ground black pepper

8 ounces (225 g) sharp Cheddar cheese, shredded

2 tablespoons (8 g) chopped fresh parsley (optional)

YIELD: 8 servings
213 calories; 17 g fat; 13 g protein; 3 g carbohydrate; trace dietary fiber per serving

TWO-CHEESE CAULIFLOWER

Reader Melissa Wright, who sent this recipe for *500 More Low-Carb Recipes*, says: "Here's a cauliflower recipe that I often make for family gatherings. I adapted it from a macaroni dish that I used to love and wanted to find a way to have again. Whenever I bring it to family functions, the dish is always empty by the time I go home, and someone always asks for the recipe. Since I'm the only low-carber in the family, I find that amusing."

Preheat oven to 350°F (180°C, or gas mark 4). Lightly coat a 2-quart baking dish with nonstick cooking spray.

Put the cauliflower florets in a microwavable casserole dish, add 2 tablespoons of water (28 ml), and cover. Microwave it for 10 to 11 minutes, or until very tender (follow the package directions if using frozen).

Whisk the egg in a large bowl. Add the cottage cheese, sour cream, salt, and pepper; mix well. Stir in the Cheddar cheese.

Remove the cauliflower from the microwave and drain thoroughly any excess water. Fold the cauliflower into the cheese mixture and gently mix well. Spoon the cauliflower mixture into the prepared baking dish. Sprinkle with chopped parsley, if desired. Bake for 30 minutes. Serve immediately.

VARIATION:
Two-Cheese Cauliflower with Poppy Seeds

Stir 2 tablespoons (17 g) of poppy seeds into the cauliflower before baking. This gives it a kind of polka-dot look and adds a subtle sophistication to the flavor.

HAZELNUT GREEN BEANS

1 pound (455 g) frozen green beans

¼ cup (34 g) hazelnuts

2 tablespoons (28 ml) olive oil

2 tablespoons (28 ml) lemon juice

Salt and ground black pepper, to taste

YIELD: 8 servings

77 calories; 6 g fat; 2 g protein; 5 g carbohydrate; 2 g dietary fiber per serving

I grew up eating green beans with almonds at holiday dinners. As an adult, I've branched out a bit. Keep in mind that green beans are a bit higher in carbs than some veggies, and watch your portions.

Put your green beans in a microwaveable casserole dish with a lid, add a couple of tablespoons (30 ml) of water and nuke on high for 7 minutes.

In the meanwhile, chop your hazelnuts. Put your big, heavy skillet over medium heat, add the olive oil, and sauté the hazelnuts till they're touched with gold and smell wonderful. Remove from the heat.

By now the microwave has beeped. Go stir your beans and give 'em another 3 to 4 minutes.

When your beans are tender-crisp, drain and add to the skillet along with the lemon juice. Toss everything together, season with salt and pepper to taste, and serve.

CUMIN MUSHROOMS

8 ounces (225 g) sliced mushrooms

1½ tablespoons (22 g) butter

1½ tablespoons (22 ml) olive oil

1 teaspoon ground cumin

¼ teaspoon ground black pepper

2 tablespoons (30 g) sour cream

YIELD: 3 servings

93 calories; 8 g fat; 2 g protein; 4 g carbohydrate; 1 g dietary fiber per serving

A simply amazing accompaniment to steak or a burger. It also makes a killer omelet filling, so you might want to make extra.

Start sautéing the mushrooms in the butter and oil in a skillet over medium-high heat.

When they've gone limp and changed color, stir in the cumin and pepper. Let the mushrooms cook with the spices for a minute or two, then stir in the sour cream. Cook just long enough to heat through, and serve.

2 slices bacon

1 pound (455 g) frozen green beans, French cut

¼ medium onion

1 tablespoon (15 ml) olive oil

1 teaspoon butter

1 teaspoon dried marjoram

¼ cup (35 g) pine nuts, toasted

2 tablespoons (28 ml) balsamic vinegar

YIELD: 8 servings

73 calories; 5 g fat; 3 g protein; 5 g carbohydrate; 2 g dietary fiber per serving

BALSAMIC GREEN BEANS WITH BACON AND PINE NUTS

What's better than bacon and pine nuts? Still, remember green beans are higher in carbs than some veggies, and stick with a ½-cup portion.

First lay your bacon on a microwave bacon rack or in a glass pie plate. Nuke it for 2 minutes on high, or until crisp. Remove from the microwave, drain, and reserve.

While the bacon's cooking, put your green beans, still frozen, in a microwavable casserole dish with a lid. Add a couple of tablespoons (30 ml) of water, cover, and when the bacon is done, put 'em in the microwave for 7 minutes on high.

Cut up your onion; you want it finely minced. Now coat your big skillet with nonstick cooking spray, put it over medium heat, and add the olive oil and butter. When the butter's melted, swirl it into the olive oil, then add the onion. Sauté for just a few minutes, till the onion is translucent. Stir in the marjoram. Turn off the heat if the beans aren't done yet—it's better than burning your onion!

When the microwave beeps, stir your green beans, and give 'em 3 more minutes. You want them tender, but not overcooked.

(If your pine nuts aren't toasted, you'll need to do that, too. Spread them in a shallow pan and give them 7 or 8 minutes at 325°F [170°C, or gas mark 3] —you want them just turning golden. A toaster oven is perfect for this—who wants to heat up the oven for a little job like this? But many stores carry pretoasted pine nuts.)

Okay, your beans are done. Drain 'em, and throw 'em in the skillet with the onion—if you've turned off the heat, turn it back on to medium-high. Stir it up. Now crumble the reserved bacon into the skillet, sprinkle the pine nuts over everything, and stir it up again. Add the balsamic vinegar, stir one more time, and serve.

4 slices bacon

8 ounces (225 g) sliced mushrooms

½ teaspoon minced garlic or 1 clove fresh garlic, minced

¼ cup (15 g) diced sun-dried tomatoes—about 10 pieces before dicing

2 tablespoons (28 ml) heavy cream

⅓ cup (33 g) shredded Parmesan cheese

YIELD: 4 servings
113 calories; 8 g fat; 6 g protein; 5 g carbohydrate; 1 g dietary fiber per serving

MUSHROOMS WITH BACON, SUN-DRIED TOMATOES, AND CHEESE

Oh, come on, you have to make this! Just looking at the ingredients in the title, you know you'll love it. Have this with a steak, and tell your friends how virtuous you are, sticking to your nutritional plan.

Chop up the bacon or snip it up with kitchen shears. Start cooking it in a large, heavy skillet over medium-high heat. As some grease starts to cook out of the bacon, stir in the mushrooms.

Let the mushrooms cook until they start to change color and get soft. Stir in the garlic and cook for 4 to 5 more minutes. Stir in the tomatoes and cream and cook until the cream is absorbed.

Scatter the cheese over the whole thing, stir it in, let it cook for just another minute, and serve.

3 slices bacon

4 cups (280 g) shredded cabbage

2 tablespoons (28 ml) cider vinegar

12 drops liquid stevia (English toffee)

YIELD: 4 servings
46 calories; 3 g fat; 2 g protein; 4 g carbohydrate; 2 g dietary fiber per serving

SWEET-AND-SOUR CABBAGE

This simple dish has a country twang and an old-fashioned feel. I like it with a pan-broiled pork shoulder steak.

In a heavy skillet, cook the bacon until crisp. Remove and drain.

Add the cabbage to the bacon grease and sauté it until tender-crisp about 10 minutes.

Stir together the vinegar and stevia. Stir this into the cabbage. Crumble in the bacon just before serving, so it stays crisp.

1 head napa cabbage

¼ cup (60 g) chili garlic paste

2 tablespoons (28 ml) soy sauce

2 teaspoons dark sesame oil

1 teaspoon salt

12 drops liquid stevia (plain)

2 tablespoons (28 ml) peanut or canola oil

2 teaspoons rice vinegar

YIELD: 4 servings

175 calories; 9 g fat; trace protein; 3 g carbohydrate; trace dietary fiber per serving

DRAGON'S TEETH

This hot stir-fried cabbage is fabulous. If you didn't think cabbage could be exciting, try this! Have the exhaust fan on or a window open when you cook this—when the chili garlic paste hits that hot oil, it may make you cough. It's worth it!

I like to cut my head of napa cabbage in half lengthwise, then lay it flat-side down on the cutting board and slice it about ½-inch (1 cm) thick. Cut it one more time, lengthwise down the middle, and then do the other half head.

Mix together the chili garlic paste, soy sauce, sesame oil, salt, and stevia in a small dish, and set by the stove.

In a wok or extra-large skillet, over the highest heat, heat the peanut or canola oil. Add the cabbage and start stir-frying. After about a minute, add the seasoning mixture and keep stir-frying until the cabbage is just starting to wilt—you want it still crispy in most places. Sprinkle in the rice vinegar, stir once more, and serve.

3 pounds (1.4 kg) asparagus, all about the same thickness

1 tablespoon (15 ml) olive oil

Salt and ground black pepper, to taste

YIELD: 10 servings

29 calories; 1 g fat; 2 g protein; 3 g carbohydrate; 1 g dietary fiber per serving

ROASTED ASPARAGUS

Reader Karen Sonderman has a large asparagus bed in her yard, the lucky stiff, so she gets a metric boatload of fresh asparagus every spring. She sent this recipe for *500 More Low-Carb Recipes*, and says that this is her very favorite way to prepare it. Julie McIntosh, who tested this recipe, says, "My seven-year-old son scarfed down almost the whole batch. I had to fight him for a sample for myself! He's never liked asparagus before, but he begged me to buy more asparagus and make this again tomorrow night! This was amazing." Julie urges you to use fresh ground coarse sea salt, or kosher salt, instead of regular table salt, along with fresh ground pepper. And let this recipe serve as a lesson: Most vegetables take well to high-temperature roasting. If you're not sure what to do with a vegetable, consider roasting it.

Preheat oven to 450°F (230°C, or gas mark 8).

Gently bend each asparagus stalk until it snaps, or breaks. Toss the part that was below the break.

Pour the olive oil into an ovenproof dish or shallow baking pan large enough to accommodate the asparagus. Add salt and pepper—freshly ground is best—to taste.

Place the asparagus in the olive oil and roll it in the oil and seasonings until it is well coated.

Place in the preheated oven and roast until just tender—5 to 7 minutes for thin spears, 8 to 10 for medium, 10 to 12 for thick.

Remove and serve immediately.

You can easily top the asparagus with favorite sauces or melt butter until golden brown and pour over the top, but it is delicious just as is! Adjust the amount of oil and seasonings for larger or smaller quantities of asparagus.

1 pound (455 g) asparagus

¼ cup (55 g) butter

2 tablespoons (15 g) chopped walnuts

1 teaspoon curry powder

½ teaspoon ground cumin

9 drops liquid stevia (English toffee)

YIELD: 3 servings

189 calories; 19 g fat; 3 g protein; 5 g carbohydrate; 2 g dietary fiber per serving

ASPARAGUS WITH CURRIED WALNUT BUTTER

What is it about asparagus? It's delectable just steamed and buttered, yet it inspires such gilding of the lily.

Snap the ends off of the asparagus where they want to break naturally. Put in a microwavable container with a lid, or use a glass pie plate and plastic wrap. Either way, add a tablespoon or two (15 to 28 ml) of water, and cover. Microwave on high for 5 minutes. Don't forget to uncover as soon as the microwave goes beep, or your asparagus will keep cooking and be limp and sad!

While that's cooking, put the butter in a medium skillet over medium heat. When it's melted, add the walnuts. Stir them around for 2 to 3 minutes, until they're getting toasty. Now stir in the curry powder, cumin, and stevia, and stir for another 2 minutes or so.

Your asparagus is done by now. Fish it out of the container with tongs, put it on your serving plates, and top with the curried walnut butter.

1 pound (455 g) asparagus

½ cup (115 g) mayonnaise

2 teaspoons soy sauce

1 teaspoon dark sesame oil

¼ teaspoon chili garlic sauce

1 scallion

YIELD: 3 servings

298 calories; 33 g fat; 3 g protein; 4 g carbohydrate; 2 g dietary fiber per serving

ASPARAGUS WITH SOY AND SESAME MAYONNAISE

Serve this with fish for a fast and elegant company meal. It's super-easy to double or even triple.

Snap the ends off the asparagus where they want to break naturally. Put them in a microwave steamer or a glass pie plate. Add a couple of table-spoons (28 ml) of water, cover, and nuke on high for 5 minutes.

In the meantime, combine everything else in your food processor with the S-blade in place and run until the scallion is pulverized.

The standard way to serve this is to give everyone a puddle of sauce to dip their asparagus in. The fancy way is to spoon the sauce into a baggie, snip a teeny bit off the corner, and pipe artistic squiggles of sauce over your plates of asparagus.

By the way, if you nuke the asparagus earlier in the day and then chill it, this makes a nice salad.

PEPPERONCINI SPINACH

1 package (10 ounces, or 280 g) frozen chopped spinach, thawed

1½ teaspoons olive oil

2 pepperoncini peppers, drained and minced

1 clove garlic

1 tablespoon (15 ml) lemon juice

YIELD: 3 servings

47 calories; 3 g fat; 3 g protein; 5 g carbohydrate; 3 g dietary fiber per serving

Pepperoncini are those little hot salad peppers you sometimes get in a Greek salad. Look for 'em in the pickle section of your grocery store. If you're skittish about hot food, be aware that these are a lot milder than a jalapeño.

Put your thawed spinach in a strainer, and either press it with the back of a spoon or actually pick it up with clean hands and squeeze it—you want all the excess water out of it.

Give your medium skillet a shot of nonstick cooking spray, put it over medium-high heat, and add the olive oil. When it's hot, add the spinach, pepperoncini, and garlic. Sauté, stirring often, for about 5 minutes. Stir in the lemon juice, let it cook another minute, and serve.

SAUTÉED SESAME SPINACH

1 tablespoon (8 g) sesame seeds

1 tablespoon (14 g) coconut oil or peanut oil

1 pound (455 g) fresh spinach

2 tablespoons (28 ml) soy sauce

YIELD: 4 servings

72 calories; 5 g fat; 4 g protein; 5 g carbohydrate; 3 g dietary fiber per serving

Spinach is native to Asia, so this preparation is a natural. It's a quick-and-easy dish that goes well as a side with a simple fish dish.

Put the sesame seeds in a small, heavy skillet over medium-high heat, and stir or shake them until they're golden brown and toasty. Remove from the heat and reserve.

If you have a wok, use it for this dish. If not, coat your large, heavy skillet with nonstick cooking spray. Either way, put the pan over high heat and add the oil. When the oil is hot, add the spinach, and stir-fry till it's just barely wilted. Stir in the soy sauce, and transfer to serving plates.

Sprinkle ¾ teaspoon of the toasted sesame seeds on each serving, and serve.

1 ounce (28 g) sliced pepperoni

2 tablespoons (30 ml) olive oil, divided

1 pound (455 g) sliced mushrooms

1 bunch scallions, sliced

2 cloves garlic, crushed

1 bag (5 ounces, or 140 g) baby spinach

Salt and ground black pepper, to taste

YIELD: 6 servings

90 calories; 7 g fat; 3 g protein; 5 g carbohydrate; 2 g dietary fiber per serving

2 medium zucchini

2 tablespoons (28 ml) olive oil

2 tablespoons (28 ml) lemon juice

½ teaspoon ground coriander

¼ teaspoon dried thyme

1 clove garlic, minced

2 tablespoons (8 g) chopped fresh parsley

YIELD: 4 servings

78 calories; 7 g fat; 1 g protein; 4 g carbohydrate; 1 g dietary fiber per serving

SAUTÉED MUSHROOMS AND SPINACH WITH PEPPERONI

Try this as a side dish, smothering a chicken breast, or as an omelet filling. I can't think of a bad way to serve this.

Slice your pepperoni into teeny strips. Heat 1 tablespoon (15 ml) of the olive oil in your large, heavy skillet, add the pepperoni, and sauté it until it's crisp. Lift out with a slotted spoon, and drain on paper towels.

Add the remaining 1 tablespoon (15 ml) oil to the skillet, and let it heat over a medium-high burner. Add the mushrooms, and sauté them until they're softened and starting to brown. Add the sliced scallions and sauté for another few minutes, until they're starting to brown, too. Stir in the garlic, then add the spinach. Turn the whole thing over and over, just until the spinach wilts. Stir in the pepperoni bits, season with salt and pepper to taste, and serve.

LEMON-HERB ZUCCHINI

Do you have any idea how low in carbs zucchini is? And it takes up flavors beautifully.

Cut your zukes in half lengthwise, then slice them ¼ inch (6 mm) thick.

Coat your large, heavy skillet with nonstick cooking spray, and put over medium-high heat. Add the olive oil. When it's hot, add your sliced zucchini, and sauté, stirring frequently, till it's just softening.

Add the lemon juice, coriander, thyme, and garlic. Stir everything together, reduce the heat to medium-low, and let it simmer for another few minutes.

Stir in the parsley just before serving.

1 cup (100 g) chopped celery

¼ cup (40 g) chopped onion

Salt and ground black pepper, to taste

Poultry seasoning, to taste

2 teaspoons Splenda

2 tablespoons (28 g) butter

¼ cup (60 ml) heavy cream

½ cup (120 ml) chicken broth

10 ounces (280 g) plain pork rinds or skins (about 3 average bags), broken into small pieces —about ½ to 1 inch

4 eggs

YIELD: 8 servings

276 calories; 18 g fat; 25 g protein; 2 g carbohydrate; trace dietary fiber per serving

PORK RIND STUFFING

My erstwhile cyber-pal, Trish Z., kindly gave permission for this recipe, remarkably similar to cornbread dressing, to appear in *500 More Low-Carb Recipes*. Though it is not so much a vegetable dish, I include it here as a great choice for holiday meals, and for all you hard-core Stove Top Stuffing fans.

Preheat oven to 325ºF (170ºC or gas mark 3).

Sauté the celery, onion, salt, pepper, poultry seasoning, sweetener, and butter in a frying pan until transparent and tender. Add the remaining ingredients and mix together until the pork rinds are coated and moist.

Put into a baking dish and bake for 35 to 50 minutes, until set like regular bread stuffing.

Feel free to add more eggs or cream to get the texture you are used to. Some people also add mushrooms, sage, sausage, or oysters.

CHAPTER 8
Poultry

Forget the hamburger; chicken is America's favorite meat. But owing to thirty years of fat-phobia, a sad thing has happened: Many people equate "chicken" with "boneless, skinless chicken breast." It's a shame. Boneless, skinless breast is bland, and often dry, requiring considerable doctoring to taste like much. It's also pricey. Really, the best thing to be said about boneless, skinless breast is that it's quick to cook.

Not only is chicken skin delicious, but it's also a great source of gelatin—healthful stuff. I recommend you enjoy it often. And bones? Save them to make broth far tastier and more nutritious than anything you can buy at the grocery store.

You'll find some new ways to cook chicken here, both on the bone and off, with skin and without. You'll also fine some turkey recipes you'll thank me for the Saturday after Thanksgiving.

**1 whole chicken, about
5 pounds (2.3 kg)**

**1 heaping tablespoon (18 g)
mayonnaise**

Salt and ground black pepper

Paprika

Onion powder

YIELD: 6 servings

600 calories; 44 g fat; 48 g protein;
1 g carbohydrate; trace dietary
fiber per serving (However, those
calorie and fat counts are high,
because MasterCook does not
calculate the fat that cooks off.)

TASTY ROASTED CHICKEN

This recipe appeared in *500 Low-Carb Recipes*. I repeat it here because few things are simpler or more satisfying than a plain roasted chicken, which is inexpensive, too! Whole chickens frequently go on sale; I stock up when they hit 99 cents per pound. And now that most people buy their chicken cut up, there's something sort of festive about a whole roasted chicken.

Preheat oven to 375ºC (190ºC, or gas mark 5).

If your chicken was frozen, make sure it's completely thawed—if it's still a bit icy in the middle, run some hot water inside it until it's not icy anymore. Take out the giblets; if you've never cooked a whole chicken before, you'll find them in the body cavity. (I usually feed them to my dogs.)

Dry your chicken with paper towels and put it on a plate. Scoop your mayonnaise out of the jar and into a small dish, being careful not to contaminate the jar. Using clean hands, give your chicken a nice mayo massage. That's right, rub that chicken all over with the mayonnaise, coating every inch of skin. Sprinkle the chicken liberally with salt, pepper, paprika, and onion powder, all four equally, on all sides. Put the chicken on a rack in a shallow roasting pan, and put in the oven. Leave the bird there for 1½ hours, or until the juices run clear when you stick a fork in where the thigh joins the body. Remove from the oven, and let the chicken sit for 10 to 15 minutes before carving, to let the juices settle.

1½ pounds (680 g) boneless, skinless chicken thighs

2 tablespoons (28 ml) lemon juice

1 tablespoon (15 ml) lime juice

1 shallot, minced

5 cloves garlic, crushed

1 tablespoon (8 g) grated fresh ginger root

2 tablespoons (28 ml) soy sauce

3 drops liquid stevia (plain)*

1 teaspoon ground turmeric

---

*Alternative Sweetener

½ teaspoon Splenda or Stevia in the Raw

YIELD: 4 servings

210 calories; 3 g fat; 40 g protein; 3 g carbohydrate; trace dietary fiber per serving

GOLDEN TRIANGLE CHICKEN KABOBS

The turmeric turns this Asian-inspired chicken a pretty color, and it tastes great, too. Did you know that turmeric has been studied for its tumor-fighting properties? Good stuff.

Cut your chicken into 1-inch (2.5 cm) cubes. This is easier if it's somewhat frozen.

Put your chicken cubes in a resealable plastic bag, then stir together everything else and pour it in. Seal the bag, pressing out the air as you go. Stash the bag in the fridge for at least several hours (24 hours is brilliant). If you're going to be using bamboo skewers, you might put them in water to soak now.

When dinnertime rolls around, preheat your broiler, or fire up your barbecue. Pull the bag out of the fridge, pour off the marinade into a small bowl, and reserve. Thread your chicken cubes onto 4 skewers.

Start your skewers grilling or broiling, giving them about 5 minutes. Baste both sides of your kabobs with that reserved marinade (discard the rest of the marinade to avoid germs), turn them over, and give them another 5 minutes, or till done through.

2 pounds (900 g) boneless, skinless chicken thighs

¼ cup (60 ml) olive oil

¼ cup (60 ml) lemon juice

2 cloves garlic, minced

2 tablespoons (7 g) red pepper flakes

Salt and ground black pepper, to taste

Fresh parsley, for garnish, if desired

1 lemon, cut into 6 wedges

YIELD: 6 servings

246 calories; 17 g fat; 22 g protein; 2 g carbohydrate; trace dietary fiber per serving

CHICKEN SKEWERS *DIAVOLO*

Italian-style chicken kabobs. How about serving this with sautéed zucchini and mushrooms?

Cut your chicken into 1-inch (2.5 cm) cubes. Put them in a big resealable plastic bag. Combine the olive oil, lemon juice, garlic, red pepper flakes, and salt and pepper, and pour over the chicken. Seal the bag, pressing out the air as you go. Turn to coat, then throw the bag in the fridge, and let the chicken marinate for at least 4 to 5 hours, and all day won't hurt a bit.

If you're going to use bamboo skewers, put them in water to soak 30 minutes before cooking time.

When cooking time comes, preheat your grill or broiler and pour off the marinade into a dish and reserve. Thread the chicken chunks onto 6 skewers. You can now grill them or broil them for about 8 minutes, or until done through (cut into a chunk to see), basting often with the reserved marinade —but stop basting with at least a couple of minutes cooking time to go, to be sure all the raw chicken germs are killed.

Garnish each skewer with a little minced parsley, if using, and serve with a lemon wedge to squeeze over it.

1 pound (455 g) ground chicken

2 tablespoons (7 g) chopped dry-pack sun-dried tomatoes, chopped fine

2 tablespoons (20 g) minced onion

1 clove garlic, minced

1 tablespoon (2.5 g) minced fresh basil (or 1 teaspoon dried)

1 teaspoon minced fresh oregano (or ¼ teaspoon dried)

1 teaspoon paprika

½ teaspoon salt or Vege-Sal

¼ teaspoon ground black pepper

¼ teaspoon cayenne

YIELD: 3 servings

345 calories; 14 g fat; 47 g protein; 5 g carbohydrate; 1 g dietary fiber per serving

CHICKEN BURGERS WITH BASIL AND SUN-DRIED TOMATOES

Sunny bright flavor; truly wonderful made with fresh herbs. You could use ground turkey, if you prefer.

Just combine everything in a mixing bowl and use clean hands to mix it all together until it's well blended. Form into 3 patties. If you've got a little time, put them on a plate, and chill them for 30 minutes before cooking.

I like to pan-broil these in my big, heavy skillet for about 5 to 6 minutes per side. Try topping them with mayonnaise with a little lemon juice and chopped basil stirred in.

5 pounds (2.5 kg) bone-in chicken thighs without skin

1½ cups (345 g) plain yogurt

¼ cup (60 ml) olive oil

2 tablespoons (16 g) grated fresh ginger root

1 tablespoon (15 ml) lemon juice

2 teaspoons chili powder

2 teaspoons ground turmeric

1 teaspoon salt or Vege-Sal

1 teaspoon ground coriander

½ teaspoon ground cumin

½ teaspoon ground cinnamon

½ teaspoon ground cloves

4 cloves garlic

2 bay leaves, whole

YIELD: 6 servings

387 calories; 20 g fat; 45 g protein; 5 g carbohydrate; 1 g dietary fiber per serving

TANDOORI CHICKEN

Okay, without an Indian tandoor oven this isn't truly authentic, but oh, my gosh, it's good. Feel free to use white meat chicken if you prefer, or a cut-up whole chicken, but do use chicken on the bone. And if you skin your own chicken, see the recipe for Chicken Chips (page 42), for what to do with the skin.

Skin the chicken if you didn't buy it that way. Put it in a nonreactive baking pan—glass or enamel are ideal, but stainless steel will do. Don't use aluminum or iron.

Put everything else in your blender, and run it until you have a smooth sauce.

Pour the sauce over the chicken, and use tongs to turn each piece to coat. Cover the baking pan with plastic wrap, slide it into the fridge, and let it sit for a minimum of 4 hours; a whole day is ideal.

Pull your chicken out of the fridge, and let it come to room temperature. Meanwhile, preheat your oven to 350ºF (180ºC, or gas mark 4).

When the oven is hot, pull the plastic wrap off the baking pan and slide it in to cook. Roast for 45 minutes to 1 hour, turning the chicken occasionally with your tongs.

1 tablespoon (6 g) ground black pepper

1 tablespoon (6 g) ground allspice

1 teaspoon dried oregano

½ teaspoon ground cumin

1 teaspoon lime juice

1 teaspoon lemon juice

3 drops orange extract

2 pounds (900 g) chicken thighs

YIELD: 4 servings

389 calories; 28 g fat; 31 g protein; 3 g carbohydrate; 1 g dietary fiber per serving

YUCATÁN CHICKEN

In the Yucatán they marinate chicken in the juice of bitter oranges. Well, I've got to tell you, those bitter oranges are mighty thin on the ground here in southern Indiana. So I've used lemon and lime juice with orange extract to get a similar flavor here.

Mix together everything but the chicken. Rub this mixture all over your chicken thighs, and even up under the skin. Refrigerate for several hours.

When cooking time comes, preheat your broiler, arrange the chicken on your broiler rack, skin-side down, and broil about 6 inches from the heat for 15 minutes or so. Turn, and give it another 10. Turn again, and give it at least another 5 minutes. Now turn a piece skin-side up, and pierce it to the bone. If the juice runs clear, it's done. If it runs pink, you need to give it a little longer.

You can also cook this on your barbecue grill if you like. Indeed, if you want to take something along to the park or the beach to grill while you're there, do the flavoring step early in the day, marinating the chicken in a big resealable plastic bag. Then grab the bag of chicken, throw it in your cooler, and go.

Serve with a big green salad.

4 boneless, skinless chicken breasts, total 1½ pounds (680 g)

1 jar (6 ounces, or 170 g) marinated artichoke hearts, drained

3 ounces (85 g) Boursin cheese (or similar spreadable garlic-herb cheese)

¼ teaspoon ground black pepper

½ tablespoon (7 g) butter

YIELD: 4 servings
298 calories; 12 g fat; 41 g protein; 4 g carbohydrate; 2 g dietary fiber per serving

CHICKEN BREASTS STUFFED WITH ARTICHOKES AND GARLIC CHEESE

Delicious and filling, this is an impressive dish that's great for dinner parties.

Preheat oven to 375ºF (190ºC, or gas mark 5).

One by one, place each chicken breast in a big, heavy resealable plastic bag, and seal it, pressing out the air as you go. Then use any heavy, blunt implement that's handy—I use a 3-pound (1.3 kg) dumbbell—to pound the chicken till it's ¼ inch (6 mm) thick all across. Repeat with all your chicken breasts.

Throw your drained artichoke hearts and your cheese in your food processor, with the S-blade in place. Add the pepper, too. Pulse until the artichokes are chopped fine, but not puréed.

Spread one-quarter of the cheese mixture on each breast, and roll up jelly-roll fashion. Hold closed with toothpicks.

Coat your large, heavy skillet with nonstick cooking spray, and put it over medium-high heat. When it's hot, add the butter, and swirl it around to cover the bottom of the skillet. Now add your chicken rolls, and sauté till they're lightly golden, about 3 minutes per side.

If your skillet's handle isn't ovenproof, wrap it in foil. Slide the whole thing into the oven, and let it bake for 15 minutes, or until done through, and serve.

CHICKEN IN CREAMY HORSERADISH SAUCE

4 pounds (1.8 kg) cut-up chicken pieces

1 tablespoon (14 g) butter

1 tablespoon (15 ml) olive oil

¾ cup (175 ml) chicken broth

1½ teaspoons chicken bouillon concentrate

1 tablespoon (15 g) prepared horseradish

4 ounces (115 g) cream cheese

¼ cup (60 ml) heavy cream

Guar or xanthan (optional)

Salt and ground black pepper, to taste

YIELD: 8 servings
442 calories; 34 g fat; 30 g protein; 1 g carbohydrate; trace dietary fiber per serving

Don't think that just because this has horseradish it's really strong—the sauce is mellow, subtle, and family friendly. Serve over Fauxtatoes (page 78) to soak up every drop.

In your big, heavy skillet, over medium-high heat, brown the chicken in the butter and olive oil. Transfer to slow cooker.

Stir together the chicken broth, bouillon concentrate, and horseradish. Pour over the chicken. Cover the pot, set the slow cooker to low, and let cook for 6 hours.

When time's up, fish out the chicken and put it on a platter. Cut the cream cheese into chunks, and melt it into the sauce, then stir in the heavy cream. Thicken with your guar or xanthan shaker if you think it needs it. Season with salt and pepper to taste, and serve.

CREAMY CHICKEN AND NOODLES IN A BOWL

1 package (8 oz or 225 g) tofu shirataki, fettuccini width

¼ cup (45 g) jarred roasted red peppers

5 kalamata olives

1 scallion

1 tablespoon (4 g) minced fresh parsley

3 tablespoons (45 g) chive-and-onion cream cheese

3 ounces (85 g) precooked chicken breast strips—mine had Southwestern seasoning

Salt and ground black pepper, to taste

YIELD: 1 serving
285 calories; 22 g fat; 16 g protein; 5 g carbohydrate; 1 g dietary fiber per serving

This is as good a make-it-in-the-bowl recipe as I've ever come up with, and it's quite filling. Takes less than 15 minutes, too.

Snip open the packet of shirataki, drain and rinse them, and throw them in a microwavable bowl. Nuke them on high for 2 minutes.

While that's happening, drain and dice your roasted red peppers.

When the microwave beeps, drain the shirataki again. Put them back in for another 2 minutes.

Pit your kalamatas—just squish them with your thumb and pick the pits out—then chop them up. Slice your scallion, including the crisp part of the green, and chop your parsley, too.

Drain your noodles one last time. Now add the cream cheese and chicken breast strips and nuke the mixture for just 30 more seconds.

When it comes out, throw in the peppers, olives, scallions, and parsley. Stir it up until the cheese melts, season with salt and pepper to taste, and devour!

2 cloves garlic, crushed

½ cup (120 ml) olive oil

1 pound (455 g) boneless, skinless chicken breast

Salt and ground black pepper, to taste

1 lemon

2 tablespoons (28 ml) water

¼ cup (10 g) minced fresh basil

2 tablespoons (8 g) minced fresh parsley

YIELD: 3 servings

508 calories, 40 g fat; 34 g protein; 5 g carbohydrate; 1 g dietary fiber per serving

LEMON-HERB CHICKEN BREAST

This dish is simple and classic and summery. With the dish at 5 grams of carbs per serving, you'll be eating this solo, but sliced ripe tomatoes would be nice for the other diners.

Put the garlic in a measuring cup and pour the olive oil over it. Let it sit.

Give a skillet a squirt of nonstick cooking spray and put it over a high burner.

Now grab your chicken and a blunt, heavy object and pound your breast out to an even ½-inch (1 cm) thickness. Cut into 3 portions and season with salt and pepper on both sides.

Pour half of the garlicky olive oil into your now-hot skillet, swirl it around, and throw in your chicken. Cover it with a tilted lid—leave a crack—and let it cook for 3 to 4 minutes.

Your chicken should be golden on the bottom now; flip it! Re-cover with the tilted lid and give it another 3 to 4 minutes. In the meantime, roll your lemon under your palm, pressing down firmly. This will help it render more juice. Slice your lemon in half and flick out the seeds with the tip of a knife.

When your chicken is golden on both sides, squeeze one of the lemon halves over it. Flip it to coat both sides, turn the burner down to medium-low, and re-cover with that tilted lid. Let it cook until it's done through.

Plate your chicken and then add the water and the juice of the other lemon half to the skillet. Stir it all around with a fork, scraping up the tasty brown bits, and then pour this over the chicken. Top with the herbs and a drizzle of the remaining garlic olive oil and then serve.

4 pounds (1.8 kg) skinless chicken thighs—I'd use bone-in

3 tablespoons (45 ml) oil

½ cup (120 ml) white wine vinegar

½ cup (120 ml) lemon juice

3 tablespoons (45 ml) brandy

1 teaspoon grated orange zest

½ teaspoon orange extract

¼ teaspoon liquid stevia (lemon drop)

8 scallions, sliced

6 ounces (170 g) cream cheese

Salt and ground black pepper, to taste

YIELD: 8 servings

384 calories; 24 g fat; 34 g protein; 4 g carbohydrate; trace dietary fiber per serving

CHICKEN IN CREAMY ORANGE SAUCE

Fruit flavors go well with chicken, but it can be a challenge to get a full, fruity flavor without all the carbs. This recipe succeeds nicely, and with slow-cooker convenience. You'll want to eat a very low-carb vegetable side or salad with this—a few asparagus spears would be lovely.

In your big, heavy skillet, over medium-high heat, brown the chicken in the oil all over. Transfer to your slow cooker.

Stir together the white wine vinegar, lemon juice, brandy, orange zest, orange extract, and stevia. Pour over the chicken. Cover the pot, set the slow cooker to low, and cook for 6 hours.

When cooking time is up, transfer the chicken to a platter. Add the sliced scallions to the liquid in the pot, then add the cream cheese, cut into chunks, and stir till it's melted. Season with salt and pepper. Serve the sauce over the chicken.

3 tablespoons (42 g) coconut oil

2 teaspoons garam masala

1 teaspoon ground cinnamon

1 teaspoon ground turmeric

½ medium onion, chopped

2 cloves garlic, crushed

1 tablespoon (8 g) grated fresh ginger root

1 teaspoon cayenne

1 can (14 fluid ounces, or 425 ml) unsweetened coconut milk

¾ cup (175 ml) chicken broth, or turkey broth, if you have it

4 cups (560 g) diced cooked turkey

Salt, to taste

YIELD: 8 servings

349 calories; 27 g fat; 23 g protein; 4 g carbohydrate; 1 g dietary fiber per serving

THANKSGIVING WEEKEND CURRY

Amazing, if I do say so myself. If you don't have any leftover turkey in the house, you could cut up a rotisserie chicken instead. You can also serve this over shirataki, if you like. Look for garam masala, an Indian spice blend, at a store with a good spice section.

In your big, heavy skillet, over medium-low heat, melt the coconut oil. Add the garam masala, cinnamon, turmeric, and stir for a minute or so.

Add the onion, and sauté until it's translucent.

Now add the garlic, ginger, and cayenne. Pour in the coconut milk and chicken broth. Stir it up until you've got a creamy sauce.

Stir in the turkey, and turn the burner to low. Let the whole thing simmer for 15 minutes or so.

Season with salt to taste and serve in bowls with soup spoons.

1 pound (455 g) frozen broccoli, thawed

1 pound (455 g) roasted turkey, sliced

1 cup (100 g) grated Parmesan, divided

1 cup (225 g) mayonnaise

1 cup (235 ml) heavy cream

2 tablespoons (28 ml) dry vermouth

YIELD: 6 servings
614 calories; 54 g fat; 31 g protein; 5 g carbohydrate; 2 g dietary fiber per serving

SUPER-EASY TURKEY DIVAN

My husband adores this! A handy recipe for the weekend after Thanksgiving. Double it and you can feed a crowd a fresh new meal with your leftovers.

Preheat oven to 350ºF (180ºC, or gas mark 4). Coat an 8-inch (20 cm) square baking dish with nonstick cooking spray.

Cover the bottom of the pan with the broccoli—I use "cut" broccoli, which is bigger than chopped broccoli but smaller than spears.

Cover the broccoli with slices of leftover turkey. I like to put the white meat on one side and the dark on the other, so people can choose.

In a mixing bowl, combine all but 2 tablespoons (10 g) of the Parmesan with the mayonnaise, cream, and vermouth. Pour over the turkey and broccoli. Sprinkle the remaining Parmesan on top. Bake until it's getting golden, about a half hour.

3 pounds (1.4 kg) boneless, skinless turkey breast (in one big hunk, not thin cutlets)

2 tablespoons (28 g) butter

¼ cup (15 g) chopped fresh parsley

2 teaspoons dried tarragon

½ teaspoon salt or Vege-Sal

¼ teaspoon ground black pepper

1 cup (70 g) sliced fresh mushrooms

¼ cup (60 ml) dry white wine

1 teaspoon chicken bouillon concentrate

Guar or xanthan (optional)

YIELD: 8 servings
281 calories; 14 g fat; 34 g protein; 1 g carbohydrate; trace dietary fiber per serving

TURKEY WITH MUSHROOM SAUCE

This takes about 3 minutes to throw together and will feed a crowd. Add to that the usual low cost of turkey, and the fact that it tastes great, and you've got a winner. I'd serve the Chicken-Almond "Rice" (page 79) with this.

In your big skillet, sauté the turkey breast in the butter till it's golden all over. Transfer to the slow cooker.

Sprinkle the parsley, tarragon, salt, and pepper over the turkey breast. Dump the mushrooms on top. Mix the wine and bouillon concentrate together until the bouillon dissolves, and pour it in as well. Cover the pot, and cook on low for 7 to 8 hours.

When it's done, fish the turkey out and put it on a platter. Transfer about half of the mushrooms to your blender, and add the liquid from the pot. Blend until mushrooms are puréed. Scoop the rest of the mushrooms into the serving dish for the sauce, add the liquid, and thicken further with your guar or xanthan shaker, if needed.

BALSAMIC-GLAZED CHICKEN AND PEPPERS

Think of this as an Italian stir-fry. And with all those vegetables, who needs a side dish?

1 pound (455 g) boneless, skinless chicken breast

½ green bell pepper

½ red bell pepper

1 small onion

2 cloves garlic, crushed

2 tablespoons (28 ml) olive oil

2 tablespoons (28 ml) balsamic vinegar

1 teaspoon Italian seasoning

YIELD: 4 servings

217 calories; 10 g fat; 26 g protein; 5 g carbohydrate; 1 g dietary fiber per serving

Cut your chicken into ½-inch (1 cm) cubes. Cut your peppers into strips— I like to cut them thinly lengthwise, then once crosswise. Cut your onion in half vertically, and slice vertically. Mince your garlic and have it standing ready, too.

Put your large, heavy skillet over medium-high heat. Add the olive oil, and let it get hot. Now throw in the chicken, peppers, and onions, and stir-fry them until all the pink is gone from the chicken, and the vegetables are starting to soften a bit.

Add the garlic, balsamic vinegar, and Italian seasoning, stir everything up. Let the whole thing cook, stirring often, until the vinegar has reduced and become a bit syrupy, then serve.

SKILLET CITRUS CHICKEN

Orange, lemon, and lime plus mustard give a tangy snap to this chicken. You'll want a very low-carb side with this. Polaner Sugar Free with Fiber preserves are the lowest in carbs I've found, and very tasty, too.

1 tablespoon (15 ml) olive oil

3 pounds (1.4 kg) chicken thighs

½ cup (120 ml) chicken broth

2 tablespoons (40 g) low-sugar orange marmalade preserves

2 tablespoons (28 ml) lemon juice

2 tablespoons (28 ml) lime juice

2 teaspoons brown mustard

18 drops liquid stevia (lemon drop)

2 cloves garlic, crushed

YIELD: 5 servings

499 calories; 36 g fat; 38 g protein; 4 g carbohydrate; trace dietary fiber per serving

Coat your large, heavy skillet with nonstick cooking spray, and put it over medium-high heat. When it's hot, add the olive oil, then the chicken, skin-side down. Sauté until the chicken is lightly golden, then turn bone-side down. Brown for another 5 minutes or so.

While that's happening, stir together the chicken broth, low-sugar marmalade, lemon juice, lime juice, mustard, stevia, and garlic. When the chicken is browned, pour the broth mixture into the skillet. Partially cover the skillet with a "tilted lid"—leave a crack of about ¼ inch (6 mm) to let some steam out. Turn the burner to low, and let the chicken simmer for 20 minutes.

When the time is up, uncover the chicken and remove it to a platter. Keep it in a warm place while you turn up the burner, and boil down the sauce until it's a little syrupy. Pour the sauce over the chicken, and serve.

3 pounds (1.4 kg) turkey roast

2 tablespoons (28 ml) oil—light olive oil or MCT oil

1 cup (100 g) cranberries

½ cup (80 g) chopped onion

¼ cup (60 g) erythritol*

3 tablespoons (33 g) spicy mustard

¼ teaspoon red pepper flakes

1 peach, peeled and chopped

---

*Alternative Sweetener

¼ cup (6 g) Splenda or ¼ cup (12 g) Stevia in the Raw

¼ teaspoon liquid stevia

12 drops EZ-Sweetz Family Size

6 drops EZ-Sweetz Travel Size

YIELD: 8 servings

255 calories; 8 g fat; 31 g protein; 4 g carbohydrate; 1 g dietary fiber per serving

CRANBERRY-PEACH TURKEY ROAST

This fruity sauce really wakes up the turkey roast!

If your turkey roast is like mine (a Butterball) it will be a boneless affair of light and dark meat rolled into an oval roast, enclosed in a net sack. Leave it in the net for cooking, so it doesn't fall apart on you. Heat the oil in your big, heavy skillet, and brown the turkey roast on all sides. Transfer it to a slow cooker.

Put the cranberries, onion, erythritol, mustard, red pepper flakes, and chopped peach in your blender, or in your food processor with the S-blade in place. Run it until you have a coarse puree. Pour this over the roast. Cover the slow cooker, set it to low, and let it cook for 6 to 7 hours.

Remove the roast to a platter and stir up the sauce. Transfer the sauce to a sauce boat to serve with the turkey. You can remove the net from the turkey before serving, if you like, but I find it easier just to use a good sharp knife to slice clear through the netting, and let each diner remove his or her own.

CHAPTER 9
Fish and Seafood

Fish and seafood are wildly popular, the darlings of restaurant menus. Yet many people shy away from cooking fish and seafood at home, afraid that anything less plebeian than fish sticks will be complicated and touchy. Happily, this is not so; fish and seafood are easy! Furthermore, they're quick, making fish and seafood a great choice when you're short on time. It's hard to come up with a fish recipe that takes more than 20 minutes to cook.

Sadly, many fish recipes, and perhaps most frozen, prepared fish dishes, are breaded or battered. I'm here to help you change that!

By the way, if you're looking for something super-simple, feel free to simply eat crab legs or lobster tail dunked in all the lemon butter you want. Some grocery stores will steam a lobster for you on demand!

Regarding that lemon butter: Since fish is naturally low in fat—even salmon gets only 28 percent of its calories from fat—it's nice to pair these dishes with a higher fat side or salad.

However, skip the fake seafood, a.k.a surimi. It has carbs added, often in startling quantities. And be wary of things like "crab dip" and "crab salad"—if they're affordable, they're probably made with surimi.

1 tablespoon (14 g) coconut oil

1½ pounds (680 g) salmon fillet, cut into 4 servings

½ cup (120 ml) vinaigrette

½ cup (120 ml) lemon juice

2½ tablespoons (4 g) Splenda, or the equivalent in liquid Splenda

2 tablespoons (28 ml) lime juice

1 teaspoon brown mustard

1 teaspoon chili powder

¼ teaspoon orange extract

YIELD: 4 servings

384 calories; 25 g fat; 34 g protein; 5 g carbohydrate; trace dietary fiber per serving

1½ pounds (680 g) salmon fillet, cut into 4 servings

¼ cup (60 g) mayonnaise

4 teaspoons (20 g) pesto sauce

4 tablespoons (20 g) shredded Parmesan cheese

YIELD: 4 servings

342 calories; 21 g fat; 37 g protein; 1 g carbohydrate; trace dietary fiber per serving

SALMON IN CITRUS VINAIGRETTE

My husband said this was perhaps the best salmon dish he'd ever had. In the interest of full disclosure, it should be stated that he's fond of salmon, my cooking, and me, and he was hungry. Still.

Coat a big skillet with nonstick cooking spray and put it over medium heat. Throw in the coconut oil and when it's melted, swirl it around and then add the salmon.

While the salmon is getting a little touch of gold, throw everything else in the blender and run the thing.

Okay, go back and flip your salmon. Let it get a little gold on the other side, too.

Add the vinaigrette mixture to the skillet and turn the burner up to medium-high. Let the whole thing cook for another 5 minutes, or until the salmon is done through.

Plate the salmon and turn up the burner. Boil the sauce hard until it's reduced and starting to get a little syrupy. Pour over the salmon and serve.

SALMON WITH PESTO MAYONNAISE

Salmon fillets are my husband's favorite last-minute supper, so I'm always looking for something new and interesting to do with them. Made with jarred pesto, this couldn't be easier.

Coat a shallow baking pan with nonstick cooking spray, and arrange your salmon fillets in it, skin-side down. Set the broiler for low heat, and broil the salmon about 4 inches (10 cm) from the heat source for 4 to 5 minutes.

Meanwhile, combine the mayonnaise and pesto sauce. When the initial broiling time is up, spread the pesto mayonnaise on the salmon. Top each serving with 1 tablespoon (5 g) Parmesan. Run back under the broiler for 1½ minutes, or until the cheese is lightly browned.

2 tablespoons (28 ml) boiling water

2 tablespoons (7 g) chopped sun-dried tomatoes

8 ounces (230 g) salmon fillet, in 2 pieces about the same shape

3 teaspoons (15 ml) olive oil, divided

¼ cup (18 g) sliced mushrooms—portobellos, the little ones

1 ounce (28 g) provolone cheese, sliced

1 teaspoon minced fresh parsley

YIELD: 2 servings
252 calories; 15 g fat; 27 g protein; 3 g carbohydrate; 1 g dietary fiber per serving

SUN-DRIED TOMATO-PORTOBELLO SALMON ROAST

My pal Julie calls this, I-can't-believe-this-could-be-diet-y dish that you would order again and again in a restaurant!" Sounds like an endorsement to me.

Preheat oven to 350ºF (180ºC, or gas mark 4).

Pour the boiling water over your chopped sun-dried tomatoes. Let them sit while you use a sharp knife to remove the skin from your salmon if it has skin.

Coat a little skillet with nonstick cooking spray, and add 2 teaspoons of the olive oil. Sauté the mushrooms until they soften and change color.

Now lay one of your slabs of salmon fillet on a sheet pan you've coated with nonstick cooking spray or lined with nonstick foil. Lay the provolone on the salmon fillet. Drain the excess water off the tomatoes, and make a layer of them. Then top with the mushrooms. Now lay the second piece of salmon on top. Pierce with a few toothpicks or skewers to keep the layers together.

Use a basting brush to brush your salmon roast with the last teaspoon of olive oil. Sprinkle on the parsley. Now slide it into the oven for 20 to 30 minutes.

Slice in half through the layers to serve.

1½ pounds (680 g) salmon fillet, cut into 4 servings

3 tablespoons (45 g) bacon grease, melted

Salt and ground black pepper, to taste

2 tablespoons (22 g) brown mustard

2 tablespoons (30 g) grated horseradish

1 tablespoon (15 g) erythritol

YIELD: 4 servings

297 calories; 16 g fat; 35 g protein; 1 g carbohydrate; trace dietary fiber per serving

GLAZED SALMON

The mustard and horseradish lend a zip to the richness of salmon. How about simple sautéed spinach with this? Be sure to read labels to find horseradish with no sugar.

You can grill this or broil it. Either way, start your cooking device heating before you do anything else. If you're using a grill, make sure it's good and clean, so your fish won't stick. Oil the grill or broiler pan.

Brush your fish on either side with bacon grease. Season lightly with salt and pepper. (If you're using bacon grease, you may want to skip the salt.)

Mix together everything else, and have it standing by.

Lay your fish on the broiler pan or grill, and give it 3 minutes. Flip and grill the other side for 3 minutes. Now brush with the glaze, turn, and coat the other side, too. Give it another minute or so, then pull off the grill and serve with any remaining glaze. (Boil the glaze for a few minutes first, to kill any germs!)

6 pollock fillets (about 1 pound, or 455 g, total)

2 tablespoons (22 g) brown mustard

2 tablespoons (30 g) prepared horseradish

4 teaspoons (20 g) Heinz Reduced Sugar Ketchup

½ teaspoon Sriracha

YIELD: 3 servings

142 calories; 2 g fat; 27 g protein; 2 g carbohydrate; trace dietary fiber per serving

DEVILED POLLOCK

Pollock is available frozen at my grocery year-round, and is invariably cheap. If you prefer, however, you can use cod. This recipe is very easy, and quite tasty.

Preheat oven to 325ºF (170ºC, or gas mark 3).

Coat a shallow baking dish with nonstick cooking spray, and lay your fillets in it.

Mix together the mustard, horseradish, ketchup, and Sriracha. Spread this mixture over the fish, coating the surface evenly.

Bake for 20 minutes, or until the fish flakes easily, and serve.

¼ cup (55 g) butter

2 pounds (900 g) flounder fillets, in 4 servings

2 lemons

⅓ cup (75 g) mayonnaise

⅓ cup (33 g) grated Parmesan cheese

4 scallions

YIELD: 4 servings

481 calories; 32 g fat; 46 g protein; 4 g carbohydrate; 1 g dietary fiber per serving

TRANSCENDENT FLOUNDER

So-called because my husband took one bite and said, "That's transcendent!" Hope you think so, too.

Turn on your broiler and arrange a rack about 4 inches (10 cm) beneath.

Put the butter in a custard cup or glass measuring cup and microwave it for a minute to melt.

Lay a piece of foil over your broiler pan and coat it with nonstick cooking spray. Cup the edges a little. Now lay out the flounder fillets. Pour the butter evenly over the fillets and use a brush or the back of a spoon to make sure they're coated all over. Halve the lemons, pick out the seeds, and squeeze the juice over the fish.

Slide the fish under the broiler. While it's cooking, mix together the mayonnaise and Parmesan.

By now your fillets should be getting close to done; it doesn't take long. If they're cooking unevenly, turn the pan and let them cook another minute. When the flounder is getting opaque and flaky, spread the mayonnaise mixture evenly over them and slide them back under the broiler.

Slice up your scallions. Then check your fish—again, if the topping is browning unevenly, turn the pan to even it out and give it another minute or two. When the topping is evenly golden, plate the fish, scatter the sliced scallion over each serving, and eat.

2 tablespoons (28 ml) dry white wine

1 tablespoon (15 ml) lemon juice

1 tablespoon (4 g) snipped fresh dill weed, or 1 teaspoon dried dill weed

12 ounces (340 g) trout fillet

Salt and ground black pepper, to taste

YIELD: 2 servings
265 calories; 11 g fat; 35 g protein; 1 g carbohydrate; trace dietary fiber per serving

POACHED TROUT WITH DILL

Simple and classic. It's hard to beat lemon and dill with fish. I think sautéed fennel would be nice with this.

In a shallow, nonreactive pan with a lid, combine the wine and lemon juice. Put over medium heat, and bring to a simmer. Stir in the dill, and lay the trout fillets skin-side up in the wine–lemon juice mixture. Turn the heat down to low, cover the pan, and set a timer for 8 minutes.

Carefully transfer the trout fillets to 2 serving plates, turning skin-side down in the process. Pour the pan liquid over them, season lightly with salt and pepper, and serve.

6 tablespoons (90 ml) lemon juice

5 tablespoons (75 ml) extra-virgin olive oil, divided

3 tablespoons (7.5 g) chopped fresh basil

3 tablespoons (12 g) chopped fresh parsley

Salt and ground black pepper, to taste

2¼ pounds (1 kg) halibut fillets, in 4 servings

3 tablespoons (9 g) chopped fresh chives

1 medium red bell pepper, sliced into rings

YIELD: 4 servings
297 calories; 15 g fat; 36 g protein; 3 g carbohydrate; 1 g dietary fiber per serving

HALIBUT WITH LEMON-HERB SAUCE

This simple dish has a bright, summery flavor, and looks beautiful on the plate. Time to plant an herb garden?

Preheat the broiler.

Put the lemon juice, 4 tablespoons (60 ml) of the olive oil, the basil, and the parsley in your food processor with the S-blade in place. Pulse until puréed. Season with salt and pepper to taste.

Brush the halibut fillets with the remaining 1 tablespoon (15 ml) oil, and season them lightly with salt and pepper. Broil for about 5 minutes per side, or until just opaque through. Transfer to serving plates. Sprinkle the chives over the fish, spoon the sauce over that, arrange the pepper rings on top, and serve.

1 pound (455 g) monkfish

1 tablespoon (6 g) grated fresh ginger root

1 tablespoon (15 g) Heinz Reduced Sugar Ketchup

2 teaspoons chili garlic paste or Sriracha

6 ounces (170 g) asparagus, thin spears

3 scallions

1 tablespoon (15 ml) peanut oil, coconut oil, or MCT oil

1 teaspoon dark sesame oil

YIELD: 4 servings

139 calories; 6 g fat; 17 g protein; 3 g carbohydrate; 1 g dietary fiber per serving

GINGERED MONKFISH

This works equally well with lobster chunks, grouper, red snapper, or any other firm-fleshed fish in place of the monkfish. It looks very nice on the plate, and can be served over a little Cauli-Rice (page 78) to complete the meal.

Use a sharp knife to remove any membrane from the monkfish, then cut into thin, flat, round slices. Reserve.

In a small dish, stir together the ginger root, ketchup, and chili garlic paste. Brush this mixture over the monkfish slices. Let it sit for 5 minutes.

In the meantime, snap the ends off the asparagus where it wants to break naturally. Cut the spears into 1-inch (2.5 cm) lengths on the diagonal. Slice your scallions, too, including the crisp part of the green.

If you've got a wok, use it for this. If not, use your large, heavy skillet, but coat it first with nonstick cooking spray. Either way, put it over high heat, and add the peanut oil.

Now add the monkfish with its sauce, the asparagus, and the scallion. Stir-fry very gently, so as not to break up the fish. Cook for about 5 minutes, or until the fish is done through and the vegetables are tender-crisp.

Drizzle in the sesame oil, toss gently to combine, and serve.

1½ tablespoons (22 ml) olive oil

3 tablespoons (45 g) pesto sauce

18 ounces (510 g) shrimp, peeled and deveined

YIELD: 4 servings

237 calories; 12 g fat; 28 g protein; 2 g carbohydrate; trace dietary fiber per serving

PESTO SHRIMP

This quick-and-easy dish uses jarred pesto to great advantage. You could sprinkle a little extra Parmesan on top if you like. Salad with Italian Vinaigrette (page 72) is the obvious accompaniment.

How easy can it get? Combine the olive oil and pesto in your large, heavy skillet, over medium-high heat. When it's hot, throw in the shrimp and sauté them until they're pink clear through. Serve with all the pesto sauce from the skillet scraped over them.

1 tablespoon (15 ml) olive oil

1 pound (455 g) shrimp, peeled and deveined

2 teaspoons lemon juice

2 teaspoons paprika

1 teaspoon ground cumin

½ teaspoon ground ginger

⅛ teaspoon cayenne, or to taste

2 cloves garlic, minced

YIELD: 3 servings

212 calories; 7 g fat; 31 g protein; 4 g carbohydrate; 1 g dietary fiber per serving

SIZZLING MOROCCAN SHRIMP

This combination of spices is wonderful and exotic. This would be a great recipe to double for an impressive yet easy company dinner.

Coat your large, heavy skillet with nonstick cooking spray, and put it over high heat. When it's hot, add the olive oil, and throw in the shrimp. Sauté, turning often, until they're just barely pink all over. Stir in the remaining ingredients, sauté another minute or so, till the shrimp are pink throughout, and serve.

½ cup (112 g) butter

¼ cup (19 g) plain pork rind crumbs

2 tablespoons (20 g) minced onion

1 tablespoon (4 g) minced fresh parsley

1 teaspoon dried oregano or 1 tablespoon (4 g) minced fresh oregano, if you have it

½ teaspoon Tabasco sauce, or to taste

4 cloves garlic, crushed

36 clams in the shell—have the store open 'em up for you

YIELD: 6 servings

225 calories; 17 g fat; 14 g protein; 3 g carbohydrate; trace dietary fiber per serving

BAKED CLAMS

My husband spoke with longing of the baked clams he and his best friend John used to eat at a Chicagoland Italian restaurant called Capri; the clams were loaded with garlic butter and topped with bread crumbs. I took on the challenge of a low-carb version. He gave the results his hearty approval.

Put everything but the clams through the food processor until the mixture is well blended. Now put a teaspoon of this mixture on each clam. Arrange in a baking pan. At this point, you may cover and refrigerate or even freeze them.

When you're ready to cook them, first let them come to room temperature. Preheat oven to 375°F (190°F, or gas mark 5) and bake for 10 minutes, then broil 4 inches (10 cm) or so from the heat for another 3 to 5 minutes, until golden. Serve hot!

8 slices bacon

2 teaspoons chili powder

1 pound (455 g) bay scallops

YIELD: 4 servings

177 calories; 7 g fat; 23 g protein; 3 g carbohydrate; trace dietary fiber per serving

CHILI-BACON SCALLOPS

Bacon-wrapped scallops are a perennial favorite, but that whole wrapping thing is a bit time-consuming for a weeknight. The easy solution: Just sauté the two together! Chili powder adds a little extra kick. You can use sea scallops if you prefer, but bay scallops, being smaller, cook faster.

This is so simple! Put your large, heavy skillet over medium heat and snip the bacon into it in bits about ¼ inch (6 mm) wide. Let that fry.

Sprinkle the chili powder all over the scallops; I sprinkled both sides and then stirred them up to make sure they were evenly seasoned.

When the bacon bits are about halfway to done, add the scallops to the skillet and spread them out in a single layer. Let them cook for about 5 minutes, turning them a few times, until they're done through and the bacon bits are crisp. Serve with the bacon bits and pour the grease over the top!

CHAPTER 10
Beef

One of the great joys of a low-carbohydrate diet is beef, wonderful beef! After years of being told that you should eat boneless, skinless chicken breast, limiting your beef consumption to dry and flavorless round, you may now order the rib eye, medium-rare, with zero guilt (assuming, of course, you skip the baked potato). Want steak and eggs for breakfast? They're back on the menu.

Eating Mexican? Go for steak fajitas, pile the guacamole and sour cream on top, grab a fork, and dig in. If someone looks at you cross-eyed, say, "What? Doctor's orders."

You will find many ways to vary beef here. But feel free to serve your steak or hamburger patty simply with salt and pepper, perhaps with a salad and a few sautéed mushrooms.

1½ pounds (680 g) rib-eye steak

1 tablespoon (15 ml) olive oil

2 shallots

½ cup (120 ml) dry red wine

½ cup (120 ml) beef stock, or ½ teaspoon beef bouillon concentrate dissolved in ½ cup (120 ml) water

1 tablespoon (15 ml) balsamic vinegar

1 tablespoon (4 g) dried thyme

1 teaspoon brown or Dijon mustard

3 tablespoons (42 g) butter

Salt and ground black pepper, to taste

YIELD: 4 servings

428 calories; 28 g fat; 35 g protein; 2 g carbohydrate; trace dietary fiber per serving

RIB-EYE STEAK WITH WINE SAUCE

This is a classic, pure mid-twentieth-century steak-house dish. And a beautiful thing it is, too.

Cook your steak in the olive oil as described in Pan-Broiled Steak (page 117).

In the meantime, assemble everything for your wine sauce—chop your shallots and combine the wine, beef stock, vinegar, thyme, and mustard in a measuring cup with a pouring lip. Whisk them together.

When the timer goes off, flip the steak and set the timer again.

When your steak is done, put it on a platter and set it in a warm place. Pour the wine mixture into the skillet and stir it around, scraping up the nice brown bits, and let it boil hard. Continue boiling your sauce until it's reduced by at least half. Melt in the butter, season with salt and pepper, and serve with your steak.

1½ pounds (680 g) sirloin steak, trimmed

⅓ cup (80 ml) lime juice

2 tablespoons (28 ml) olive oil

¼ teaspoon ground black pepper

½ Anaheim chile pepper

2 cloves garlic

YIELD: 4 servings

415 calories; 30 g fat; 32 g protein; 3 g carbohydrate; trace dietary fiber per serving (Since you won't consume all the marinade, this count is actually a bit high.)

SIRLOIN WITH ANAHEIM-LIME MARINADE

This has a mild Southwestern feel, but an Anaheim won't take the top of your head off. A quarter of an avocado, sliced, with a squeeze of lime juice, would be perfect with this.

Put your steak in a shallow, nonreactive pan—glass or stainless steel are good—that just fits it, and pierce it all over with a fork.

Put everything else in your food processor with the S-blade in place, and run it till the pepper and garlic are pureed. Pour the marinade over the steak. Let the whole thing sit for at least a half an hour, and an hour or two is great.

Preheat the broiler or grill. Remove the steak from the marinade, reserving the marinade. Broil or grill your steak, close to high heat, until done to your liking. Baste both sides with the marinade when turning the steak over, then quit—you want the heat to kill any germs before your steak is done.

Let your steak rest for 5 minutes before carving and serving.

2 pounds (900 g) sirloin steak, trimmed, at least 1¼ inches (3 cm) thick

2 tablespoons (28 ml) soy sauce

1 tablespoon (15 ml) lime juice

2 teaspoons grated fresh ginger root

1 teaspoon ground turmeric

1 teaspoon ground black pepper

2 cloves garlic, crushed

12 drops liquid stevia (plain)*

---

*Alternative Sweeteners

2 teaspoons Splenda or Stevia in the Raw

2 drops EZ-Sweetz Family Size

1 drop EZ-Sweetz Travel Size

YIELD: 6 servings

315 calories; 21 g fat; 28 g protein; 2 g carbohydrate; trace dietary fiber per serving (You won't consume all the marinade, so consider this count a little high.)

JAKARTA STEAK

Indonesian seasonings give this steak an unusual twist. As with so many steak marinades, you can add a teaspoon of meat tenderizer to this, and use it to render an inexpensive piece of chuck fit for the grill.

I like to marinate this in a shallow, nonreactive container—glass, microwavable plastic, or enamelware. It's easier than finding a resealable plastic bag big enough for your steak. Lay the steak in the container. Now mix together everything else, pour it over the steak, and turn the steak once or twice to coat both sides. Stick it in the fridge, and let it marinate for several hours—overnight is brilliant.

You can grill this on your barbecue grill, or you can broil it. If you want to use charcoal, get it started a good 30 minutes before cooking time. Either way, grill or broil it close to the heat, to your desired degree of doneness, basting both sides with the marinade when you turn it.

Let your steak rest for 5 minutes before carving and serving. If you like, you can boil the remaining marinade hard for a few minutes to kill germs, then spoon just a little over each serving.

12 ounces (340 g) well-marbled steak—such as sirloin, T-bone, or rib eye—½ to ¾ inch (1 to 2 cm) thick

4 teaspoons (8 g) coarse cracked black pepper, divided

1 tablespoon (14 g) butter

1 tablespoon (15 ml) olive oil

2 tablespoons (28 ml) Cognac or other brandy

2 tablespoons (28 ml) heavy cream

Salt, to taste

YIELD: 2 servings
557 calories; 42 g fat; 32 g protein; 3 g carbohydrate; 1 g dietary fiber per serving

1½ pounds (680 g) steak, 1 inch (2.5 cm) thick—preferably rib eye, T-bone, sirloin, or strip

1 tablespoon bacon grease (15 g) or olive oil (15 ml)

YIELD: 4 servings
403 calories; 33 g fat; 24 g protein; 0 g carbohydrate; 0 g dietary fiber per serving

STEAK AU POIVRE WITH BRANDY CREAM

For pepper lovers only! This is one of those throwback dishes that reminds you of just how great food was before people feared fat.

Place your steak on a plate, and scatter 2 teaspoons of the pepper evenly over it. Using your hands or the back of a spoon, press the pepper firmly into the steak's surface. Turn the steak over, and do the same thing to the other side with the remaining pepper. Place a large, heavy skillet over high heat, and add the butter and olive oil. When the skillet is hot, add your steak. For a ½-inch (1 cm) thick steak, 4½ minutes per side is about right, go maybe a minute more for a ¾-inch (2 cm) thick steak.

When the steak is done on both sides, *turn off the burner*, pour the Cognac over the steak, and flame it. When the flames die down, remove the steak to a serving platter, and pour the cream into the skillet. Stir it around, dissolving the meat juices and brandy into it. Season lightly with salt, and pour over the steak.

PAN-BROILED STEAK

This is a method rather than a recipe, but it's become my favorite way of cooking a steak. It's quicker than broiling and makes a nicer crust. Don't worry about the measurements much, by the way; I just included them because they were needed for a nutritional breakdown. You know steak's got no carbs, so don't worry.

Put your large, heavy skillet—cast iron is best—over highest heat and let it get good and hot. In the meantime, you can season your steak if you like. I like the popular Montreal steak seasoning. Instead, you could top the finished steak with Bacon Butter (page156), Blue Cheese Steak Butter (page 156), or sautéed mushrooms. Or you can go for classic simplicity and just use salt and pepper.

When the skillet's hot, add the bacon grease or oil, swirl it around, and then throw in your steak. Set a timer for 5 or 6 minutes—your timing will depend on your preferred doneness and how hot your burner gets, but on my stove, 5 minutes per side with a 1-inch (2.5 cm) thick steak comes out medium-rare. When the timer goes off, flip the steak and set the timer again. When time is up, let the steak rest on a platter for 5 minutes before devouring.

6 ounces (170 g) ground chuck, in a patty

1 tablespoon (8 g) crumbled blue cheese

1 teaspoon finely minced sweet red onion

YIELD: 1 serving

511 calories; 40 g fat; 34 g protein; 1 g carbohydrate; trace dietary fiber per serving

BLEU BURGER

When I first went low carb, no-sugar-added ketchup was hard to come by. I started topping my burgers this way, and it's still a favorite.

Cook the burger by your preferred method. When it's almost done to your liking, top with the blue cheese and let it melt. Remove from the heat, put on a plate, and top with the onion.

1½ pounds (680 g) ground chuck, in 4 patties (6 ounces, or 170 g, each)

2 tablespoons (28 g) butter or (30 ml) olive oil

½ cup (80 g) sliced onion

½ cup (35 g) sliced mushrooms

⅛ teaspoon anchovy paste

1 dash soy sauce

YIELD: 4 servings

508 calories; 41 g fat; 31 g protein; 2 g carbohydrate; trace dietary fiber per serving

SMOTHERED BURGERS

Mmm … mushrooms and onions! Add a little grilled asparagus, and you have a super-quick gourmet meal.

Start cooking your burgers by your preferred method. While that's happening, melt the butter in a small, heavy skillet over medium-high heat. Add the onion and mushrooms and sauté until the onion is translucent. Stir in the anchovy paste and soy sauce. Serve the onion-mushroom mixture over the burgers.

6 ounces (170 g) ground chuck, in a patty ½ inch (1 cm) thick

1 tablespoon (6 g) coarse cracked pepper

1 tablespoon (14 g) butter

2 tablespoons (28 ml) dry white wine or dry sherry

YIELD: 1 serving

587 calories; 47 g fat; 31 g protein; 4 g carbohydrate; 2 g dietary fiber per serving

POOR MAN'S POIVRADE

A real peppery bite—not for the timid! These instructions are for a single serving, but of course you can double, triple, even quadruple this easily, depending on the size of your skillet.

Roll your raw beef patty in the pepper until it's coated all over. Fry the burger in the butter over medium heat, until done to your liking. Remove the hamburger to a plate. Add the wine to the skillet, and stir it around for a minute or two, until all the nice brown crusty bits are scraped up. Pour this over the hamburger, and serve.

¾ pound (340 g) ground beef

¾ pound (340 g) Italian sausage

⅓ cup (55 g) minced onion

2 teaspoons Italian seasoning or dried oregano

1 clove garlic, crushed

1 cup (245 g) no-sugar-added pizza sauce

3 tablespoons (15 g) grated Parmesan or Romano cheese (optional)

8 ounces (225 g) shredded mozzarella cheese

YIELD: 6 servings

527 calories; 44 g fat; 27 g protein; 5 g carbohydrate; 1 g dietary fiber per serving

MEATZA!

Here's a dish for all you pizza lovers, and I know you are legion! Add a salad, and you've got a supper that will please the whole family. No-sugar-added pizza sauce is out there, you just have to look for it (Ragu and Muir Glen make varieties that fit the bill, just check the labels to be sure). Pay attention to the Italian sausage, too. It generally has a little sugar added; choose the lowest carb.

Preheat oven to 350°F (180°C, or gas mark 4).

In a large bowl, with clean hands, combine the beef and sausage with the onion, Italian seasoning, and garlic. Mix well. Pat this out in an even layer in a 9 × 12-inch (23 × 30 cm) baking pan. Bake for 20 minutes.

When the meat comes out, it will have shrunk a fair amount, because of the grease cooking off. Pour off the grease. Spread the pizza sauce over the meat. Sprinkle the Parmesan on the sauce, if you like, and then distribute the shredded mozzarella evenly over the top. Set your broiler to high.

Put your Meatza! 4 inches (10 cm) below the broiler. Broil for about 5 minutes, or until the cheese is melted and starting to brown.

1½ pounds (680 g) lean ground beef

½ cup (80 g) finely diced onion

1 package (10 ounces, or 280 g) frozen chopped spinach, thawed and drained

8 ounces (225 g) cream cheese, softened

½ cup (120 ml) heavy cream

½ cup (50 g) shredded Parmesan cheese

Salt and ground black pepper, to taste

YIELD: 6 servings

544 calories; 46 g fat; 27 g protein; 5 g carbohydrate; 2 g dietary fiber per serving

BURGER SCRAMBLE FLORENTINE

Everyone needs a good skillet supper recipe! The only name I have to attribute this to is "Dottie," which is too bad, because my sister, who tested this recipe, says it's great.

Preheat oven to 350°F (180°C, or gas mark 4).

In a large ovenproof skillet, brown the ground beef and onion.

Add the spinach and cook through until the meat is done. Add the cream cheese, heavy cream, Parmesan, and salt and pepper to taste. Mix well, then spread evenly in the skillet.

Bake, uncovered, for 20 minutes or until bubbly and browned on top.

1½ pounds (680 g) ground beef

1 package (10 ounces, or 280 g) frozen chopped spinach, thawed

1 medium onion

2 cloves garlic

6 eggs

Salt and ground black pepper, to taste

⅓ cup (35 g) shredded Parmesan cheese

YIELD: 6 servings

406 calories; 29 g fat; 29 g protein; 5 g carbohydrate; 2 g dietary fiber per serving

JOE

My favorite one-dish skillet supper. Quick, easy, and flexible, too. Don't worry if you use a little less or a little more beef, or one more or less egg. It'll be fine!

In your large, heavy skillet over medium heat, start browning and crumbling the ground beef. While that's happening, drain the spinach well, chop the onion, and crush the garlic.

When the ground beef is half done, add the onion and garlic, and cook until the beef is done through. Pour off the extra fat if you like. Now stir the spinach into the beef. Let the whole thing cook for maybe 5 minutes.

Now, mix up the eggs well with a fork, and stir them into the beef mixture. Continue cooking and stirring over low heat for a couple of minutes, until the eggs are set. Season with salt and pepper to taste, and serve topped with the Parmesan.

PEPPERONCINI BEEF

2 to 3 pounds (0.9 to 1.4 kg) boneless chuck pot roast

1 cup (120 g) pepperoncini peppers, with the vinegar they're packed in

½ medium onion, chopped

Guar or xanthan

Salt and ground black pepper, to taste

YIELD: 6 servings (assuming a 2-pound /[0.9 kg] roast)

325 calories; 24 g fat; 24 g protein; 3 g carbohydrate; trace dietary fiber per serving

Pepperoncini are hot-but-not-scorching pickled Italian salad peppers. You'll find them in the same aisle as the olives and pickles. They make this beef very special.

Put the beef in the slow cooker, pour the pepperoncini on top, and strew the onion over that. Put on the lid, set the slow cooker to low, and leave it for 8 hours.

When it's done, transfer the meat to a platter, and use a slotted spoon to fish out the peppers and pile them on top of the roast. Thicken the juices in the pot just a little with the guar or xanthan, season with salt and pepper to taste, and serve with the roast.

ZUCCHINI MEAT LOAF ITALIANO

2 medium zucchini, chopped—about 1½ cups (185 g)

1 medium onion, chopped

2 cloves garlic, crushed

Olive oil—a few tablespoons (40 to 60 ml) or as needed

1½ pounds (680 g) ground chuck

¾ cup (75 g) grated Parmesan cheese

3 tablespoons (45 ml) olive oil

2 tablespoons (8 g) snipped fresh parsley

1 teaspoon salt

½ teaspoon ground black pepper

1 egg

YIELD: 5 servings

521 calories; 41 g fat; 31 g protein; 5 g carbohydrate; 1 g dietary fiber per serving

This is a meat loaf fit to serve to company! I adapted this from a recipe for a "zucchini mold" in a terrific Italian cookbook. It contained just a little beef. I thought, "How could more meat hurt?" I was right. It's wonderful this way, and very moist and flavorful. Note that this contains 5 grams of carbs per serving, so this counts as both your meat and your vegetable.

By the way, if you'd like to cut the cooking time in half, cook this in a muffin tin, and call it Meat Muffins.

Preheat the oven to 350ºF (180ºC, or gas mark 4).

Sauté the zucchini, onion, and garlic in the olive oil for about 7 to 8 minutes. Let it cool a bit, then put it in a big bowl with the rest of the ingredients.

Using clean hands, mix thoroughly. This will make a rather soft mixture—you can put it in a big loaf pan if you like, or form it on a broiler rack. I form it on a broiler rack because I like the grease to drip off, but keep in mind if you do it this way that you won't get it to stand very high—about 2 inches (5 cm) thick. Bake for 75 to 90 minutes, or until the juices run clear, but it's not dried out.

3 pounds (1.4 kg) beef stew meat in 1-inch (2.5 cm) cubes

3 tablespoons (45 ml) olive oil

2 cups (200 g) sliced celery

4 cloves garlic

1 teaspoon salt or Vege-Sal

¼ teaspoon ground cinnamon

¼ teaspoon ground cloves

¼ teaspoon ground black pepper

⅛ teaspoon ground allspice

⅛ teaspoon ground nutmeg

1 can (14½ ounces, or 410 g) diced tomatoes

½ cup (120 ml) dry red wine

YIELD: 8 servings
369 calories; 17 g fat; 44 g protein; 5 g carbohydrate; 1 g dietary fiber per serving

ROMAN STEW

A break from the usual Italian seasonings. This is adapted from a historic Roman stew recipe using spices from the Far East. Unusual and wonderful.

In your big, heavy skillet, over medium-high heat, brown the beef in the oil, working in a few batches. Transfer to a slow cooker.

Add the celery and garlic, then sprinkle the seasonings over everything. Now pour the canned tomatoes and the wine over everything. Cover the pot, set the slow cooker to low, and cook for 7 to 8 hours. You can thicken the pot juices a little if you like, but it's not really necessary.

2 pounds (900 g) beef round, cut into 1-inch (2.5 cm) cubes

1 large onion, chopped

2 cans (6 ½ ounces, or 184 g, each) sliced mushrooms

1½ cups (355 ml) beef broth

2 teaspoons Worcestershire sauce

1 teaspoon beef bouillon concentrate

1 teaspoon paprika

8 ounces (225 g) cream cheese

8 ounces (225 g) sour cream

YIELD: 8 servings
413 calories; 31 g fat; 28 g protein; 5 g carbohydrate; 1 g dietary fiber per serving

(NS) BEEF STROGANOFF

This creamy gravy is fabulous! Noodles are traditional with stroganoff. You could serve this on tofu shirataki fettuccine, but you'd need to cut your portion a bit to allow for another gram or two of carbs from the noodles.

Put the beef in your slow cooker. Put the onion on top, then dump in the mushrooms, liquid and all.

Mix the beef broth with the Worcestershire sauce, bouillon concentrate, and paprika, and pour over everything.

Cover and cook on low for 8 to 10 hours.

When ready to serve, cut the cream cheese into cubes, and stir into the mixture in the slow cooker until melted. Stir in the sour cream, and serve.

2 pounds (900 g) beef chuck

2 tablespoons (28 ml) olive oil

½ cup (120 ml) beef broth

1 tablespoon (18 g) beef bouillon concentrate

¾ teaspoon lemon pepper

½ teaspoon dried oregano

½ teaspoon garlic powder

¼ teaspoon onion powder

12 drops liquid stevia*

Salt and ground black pepper, to taste

---

*Alternative Sweeteners

2 teaspoons Splenda or Stevia in the Raw

2 drops EZ-Sweetz Family Size

1 drop EZ-Sweetz Travel Size

YIELD: 6 servings

364 calories; 28 g fat; 25 g protein; 1 g carbohydrate; trace dietary fiber per serving

(NS) EASY ITALIAN BEEF

This recipe originally called for an envelope of Italian salad dressing mix. Turns out that sugar is the first ingredient. So I looked up a few clone recipes and worked out the seasonings needed, and this is the result. Lemon pepper has a tiny bit of sugar in it, hence the "Next Step" classification. But this is low carb enough that you can have a crisp green salad alongside.

Trim the beef of all outside fat. Heat the oil in your big, heavy skillet over medium-high heat, and brown the beef on both sides. Transfer it to your slow cooker.

In the skillet, mix together everything else but the final salt and pepper, scraping up the nice brown stuff, so it dissolves. Pour this over the beef, cover the pot, and set the slow cooker to low. Cook for 6 to 8 hours.

When cooking time is up, season with salt and pepper to taste.

CHAPTER 11

Pork and Lamb

Probably owing to ancient taboos, pork has a bad reputation it doesn't deserve. It's nutritious stuff, an especially good source of niacin and potassium. Yes, potassium. Your average pork chop has as much potassium as a banana, and I, personally, would rather have the pork chop.

Sadly, the low-fat frenzy of the past few decades has led to pigs being bred to be leaner and leaner, rendering too many cuts of pork dry and bland. This needn't worry us! We can eat the succulent, fatty bits, like shoulder and spareribs, with zero guilt. That these are also the inexpensive cuts is a bonus.

As for lamb, I puzzle over its status in this country. It's hugely popular in the rest of the world, yet many Americans have never even tried it. I grew up on lamb—lamb chops for a quick supper, roast leg of lamb for Sunday dinner, even lamb kidneys now and then. I love the stuff.

However, lamb can be pricey. I wait till whole legs of lamb go on sale, buy one, and have the Nice Meat Guys slice it into steaks for me. These lamb steaks are cheaper and meatier than chops, quick and easy to cook, and take to a wide variety of seasonings. If you're a lamb fan, you'll find some new ideas here. If you're on the fence, remember that gyros are made of lamb, and who doesn't love gyros?

3 pounds (1.4 kg) Boston butt pork roast

2 teaspoons sea salt

1 tablespoon (15 ml) liquid smoke flavoring

1 head cabbage

¼ medium onion

YIELD: 8 servings

384 calories; 27 g fat; 33 g protein; 1 g carbohydrate; trace dietary fiber per serving

KALUA PIG WITH CABBAGE

This recipe comes first for a very good reason: It is hands down the cheapest, the easiest, and the best thing I know how to make in a slow cooker. Plus, it will feed a crowd. If you have a really huge slow cooker, feel free to scale up the recipe. By the way, that's not "Kahlua," like the coffee liqueur, it's the slow cooker adaptation of a traditional Hawaiian dish.

Take a carving fork, and stab your butt roast viciously all over. Do your best slasher movie imitation. You're making lots of holes to let the smoky flavor in.

Now sprinkle the salt all over the roast, hitting every bit of the surface, and rub it in a little. Do the same with the smoke flavoring.

Place your roast, fat-side up, in your slow cooker, cover it, set it to low, and forget about it for a good 7 to 8 hours, minimum. Then flip the roast, re-cover, and forget about it for another 7 to 8 hours.

About 1 to 1½ hours before serving time, chop your cabbage fairly coarsely and mince your onion.

Haul out your pork—it will fall apart and smell like heaven—put it in a big bowl, and shred it with a fork. Scoop out a bit of the liquid from the pot to moisten the meat if it seems to need it. Then keep it somewhere warm (or you can rewarm it later in the microwave).

Throw the cabbage and onion in the remaining liquid and toss it to coat. Cover the pot, set the slow cooker on high, and let it cook for at least an hour—you want it wilted but still a little crunchy.

Serve the meat and cabbage together.

1 tablespoon (15 ml) olive oil

12 ounces (340 g) pork loin chops (2 thin-cut chops)

¼ cup (40 g) minced onion

1 clove garlic, crushed

¼ cup (60 ml) chicken broth

1½ tablespoon (22 g) erythritol

1 tablespoon (15 ml) bourbon

5 drops maple extract

YIELD: 2 servings

225 calories; 12 g fat; 22 g protein; 2 g carbohydrate; trace dietary fiber per serving

BOURBON-MAPLE GLAZED PORK CHOPS

This quick-and-easy dish is the kind of thing you would gladly pony up for at a good restaurant. Fauxtatoes (page 78) are a great side dish here. I use Boyajian brand maple extract; I got it through Amazon.com.

Coat your large, heavy skillet with nonstick cooking spray, and put it over medium-high heat. Add the oil, and swirl it around to coat the bottom of the skillet. When the whole thing is hot, throw in your chops, and brown them on both sides, about 5 minutes per side.

Remove the chops from the skillet, and turn the heat down to medium-low. Add the onion and garlic, and sauté in the residual fat for a minute. Add the broth, erythritol, bourbon, and maple extract. Stir this around with your spatula, scraping up all the yummy brown bits stuck to the skillet.

Throw the chops back into the skillet. Turn the heat down to low, and set a timer for 3 minutes. When it goes off, flip the chops, and set the timer for another 3 minutes. By this time, the liquid should have cooked down and become syrupy.

Put the chops on serving plates, and scrape the glaze with the bits of onion and garlic over them, then serve.

1 pound (455 g) boneless pork loin, cut into 3 portions, about ¾ inch (2 cm) thick

2 ounces (55 g) Camembert cheese

1 tablespoon (14 g) butter

3 tablespoons (45 ml) dry white wine, or better yet, hard cider

1 tablespoon (2.5 g) chopped fresh sage

⅓ cup (77 g) sour cream

1½ teaspoons Dijon mustard

Ground black pepper, to taste

YIELD: 3 servings

333 calories; 20 g fat; 32 g protein; 2 g carbohydrate; trace dietary fiber per serving

PORK WITH CAMEMBERT SAUCE

This sauce is to die for, and the cheese and sour cream add fat to the very lean pork loin. Pair with a tossed green salad with vinaigrette, for contrast.

One at a time, put the pieces of pork loin in a heavy resealable plastic bag, and pound with any handy blunt object until the meat is ½ inch (1 cm) thick. (No, it's not better to just cut them to that thickness to begin with; pounding tenderizes the meat.)

Using a very sharp, thin-bladed knife, cut the rind off your Camembert as thinly as possible, to leave as much of the actual cheese as you can. Cut the cheese into ½-inch (1 cm) chunks, and reserve.

Coat your large, heavy skillet with nonstick cooking spray, and put it over medium-high heat. Add the butter. When the butter is melted and the pan is good and hot, swirl the butter around the bottom of the skillet, then lay your pork in it. Cook until lightly golden on both sides, but no more—it's easy to dry out boneless pork loin. Put the pork on a plate, and keep in a warm place.

Add the wine to the skillet, and stir it around with a spatula, scraping up all the flavorful brown bits. Add the sage, and stir again. Turn the heat down to medium-low. Now throw in those chunks of Camembert. Use your spatula to stir them around, and cut the chunks into smaller bits, until the cheese has completely melted. Whisk in the sour cream and mustard, season with pepper to taste, and it's done.

2 tablespoons (22 g) brown mustard, divided

1½ pounds (680 g) boneless pork shoulder steaks (4 steaks, about ½ inch [1 cm] thick)

1 large red onion, sliced thin

1½ tablespoons (22 ml) olive oil

1 tablespoon (15 ml) balsamic vinegar

YIELD: 4 servings

369 calories; 29 g fat; 23 g protein; 4 g carbohydrate; 1 g dietary fiber per serving

MUSTARD-GRILLED PORK WITH BALSAMIC ONIONS

I originally wrote this to use an electric tabletop grill, and it works great that way. But if you've abandoned yours, you can do the pork in your skillet instead, before you cook the onions (or in a second skillet). Use an extra tablespoon (15 ml) or so of olive oil.

Preheat your electric tabletop grill. Spread 2 teaspoons of the mustard on one side of the pork steaks, flip them, and spread another 2 teaspoons on the other side. Grill for about 5 minutes, or until done through.

While that's happening, put your big, heavy skillet over medium-high heat, and start sautéing the onion in the olive oil. Forget about tender-crisp—you want your onion soft, and turning brown. When good and caramelized, stir in the balsamic vinegar. Set aside.

By now your pork is done. Spread the remaining 2 teaspoons mustard on the pork (an extra ½ teaspoon on each piece), divide the balsamic-onions mixture among the steaks, and serve.

2 tablespoons (28 g) butter, divided

1 pound (455 g) boneless pork loin, cut into 4 servings

1 small onion, sliced

½ cup (120 ml) dry red wine

½ teaspoon beef bouillon concentrate

1 clove garlic, minced

¼ cup (30 g) chopped walnuts

¼ cup (15 g) chopped fresh parsley

YIELD: 4 servings

322 calories; 21 g fat; 23 g protein; 4 g carbohydrate; 1 g dietary fiber per serving

PORK LOIN WITH RED WINE AND WALNUTS

Elegantly understated. This is another dish that you could serve to company, with no one thinking "diet." With this dish at 4 grams of carbohydrate per serving, you'll want to choose your side dish with an eye to a very low carb count.

Coat your large, heavy skillet with nonstick cooking spray, and put it over medium-high heat. When it's hot, add 1 tablespoon (14 g) of the butter, swirl it around as it melts, then lay the pork in the skillet. Sauté until it's just golden on both sides. Remove the pork from the skillet, but keep it nearby.

Add half of the remaining butter to the skillet, and let it melt. Add the onion and sauté until it's getting limp. Spread the onion in an even layer in the skillet, and lay the pork on top.

Mix together the wine, beef bouillon concentrate, and garlic. Pour it over the pork, cover the pan with a tilted lid (leave a ¼-inch [6 mm] gap for steam to escape), turn the burner to low, and let the whole thing simmer for 20 minutes.

In the meantime, melt the remaining 1½ teaspoons butter in a small skillet over medium heat, and stir the walnuts in it for 5 minutes, until they smell a little toasty. Remove from the heat and reserve.

When the timer beeps, add the parsley to the skillet. Let the whole thing simmer for another 5 minutes or so. Serve with the pan juices and a tablespoon (7.5 g) of walnuts on each serving.

12 ounces (340 g) pork chops (2 chops, about ¾ inch [2 cm] thick)

2 tablespoons (28 ml) soy sauce

2 teaspoons grated fresh ginger root

1½ teaspoons dry sherry

1 tablespoon (14 g) coconut oil

YIELD: 2 servings

337 calories; 24 g fat; 27 g protein; 2 g carbohydrate; trace dietary fiber per serving

TOKYO GINGER PORK CHOPS

Pork chops with a Japanese accent. How about serving the Japanese Fried "Rice" (page 79) with this?

Lay your chops in a shallow nonreactive container—a glass pie plate is great. Mix together the soy sauce, ginger, and sherry, and pour over the chops, turning them once to coat. Let them marinate for 15 to 20 minutes.

Coat your large, heavy skillet with nonstick cooking spray, and put it over medium-high heat. Let it get good and hot, then add the coconut oil. Swirl it around the bottom of the skillet to cover. Now pick up your chops, let the marinade drip off (reserve the marinade), then throw 'em in the skillet. Brown them a bit on both sides, about 5 minutes each.

Pour the reserved marinade over the chops, turn the burner down, and let the chops simmer another 5 to 8 minutes, or until done through, then serve, scraping all the pan juices over them.

2 pounds (900 g) pork shoulder steaks, no more than ½ inch (1 cm) thick

Salt and ground black pepper, to taste

1 tablespoon (15 ml) olive oil

¼ cup (60 ml) chicken broth or ¼ teaspoon chicken bouillon concentrate dissolved in ¼ cup (60 ml) water

1 tablespoon (15 g) erythritol

1 tablespoon (11 g) spicy brown or Dijon mustard

5 drops maple extract

YIELD: 4 servings

437 calories; 34 g fat; 30 g protein; 1 g carbohydrate; trace dietary fiber per serving

MUSTARD-MAPLE GLAZED PORK STEAK

I rarely tire of pork steaks with just a little Cajun seasoning or barbecue rub, but this is very little extra trouble and seriously tasty. I'd probably serve coleslaw with this, but then I like coleslaw with anything.

Give your large, heavy skillet a shot of nonstick cooking spray and start it heating over high heat while you season the pork steaks with salt and pepper. In a minute or so, add the olive oil, swirl it around to coat the pan, and throw in your steaks. Cover them with a tilted lid.

Mix together everything else and place by the stove.

After about 5 minutes, flip your pork steaks and let them cook on the other side, again with a tilted lid.

When your pork steaks are almost done through, transfer them to a plate. Pour the mustard-maple mixture into the pan and stir it around, scraping up any tasty brown bits. Let it boil hard until it cooks down by about half. Put the steaks back in, flip them to coat, and let the whole thing keep cooking just a minute more until the sauce is the consistency of half-and-half. Plate the steaks, pour the sauce over them, and serve.

2 pounds (900 g) pork shoulder steaks or pork chops, no more than ½ inch (1 cm) thick

1 tablespoon bacon grease (15 g) or coconut oil (14 g)

¼ cup (60 g) erythritol

2 teaspoons spicy brown mustard

2 or 3 chipotle chiles canned in adobo with 1½ teaspoons of the sauce

2 cloves garlic, crushed

6 drops maple extract

YIELD: 4 servings
412 calories; 31 g fat; 32 g protein; 1 g carbohydrate; 1 g dietary fiber per serving

MAPLE-CHIPOTLE GLAZED PORK STEAKS

There's something about the New England–Mexican hybrid of maple and chipotle that is simply extraordinary. That this takes no more than 20 minutes is a bonus.

Put your large, heavy skillet over medium-high heat and start the pork steaks browning in the bacon grease.

Throw everything else in your blender or food processor and run until the chipotles and garlic are pulverized.

When your steaks are browned on both sides, add the glaze to the skillet and flip the steaks to coat on both sides. Cover with a tilted lid and let it cook until the steaks are done through and the glaze has cooked down a little—probably 10 minutes. Serve, scraping all the glaze from the skillet over the steaks.

3 pounds (1.4 kg) country-style pork ribs

⅔ cup (160 g) erythritol

¼ cup (40 g) chopped onion

¼ cup (60 ml) chicken broth

2 tablespoons (28 ml) soy sauce

½ teaspoon ground cinnamon

½ teaspoon ground ginger

½ teaspoon ground allspice

¼ teaspoon ground black pepper

⅛ teaspoon cayenne

⅛ teaspoon maple extract

3 cloves garlic, crushed

YIELD: 6 servings
383 calories; 29 g fat; 27 g protein; 2 g carbohydrate; trace dietary fiber per serving

MAPLE-SPICE COUNTRY-STYLE RIBS

The recipe tester who tried this recipe raved. He said it was shaping up to be the recipe by which all other recipes are judged!

Put the country-style ribs in your slow cooker. Mix together everything else, and pour over the ribs. Cover, and cook on low for 9 hours.

3 cloves garlic, divided

4 tablespoons (60 ml) olive oil, divided

3 pounds (1.4 kg) pork spareribs

1 tablespoon (7 g) paprika—smoked paprika is best

1 teaspoon ground cumin

1 teaspoon dried oregano

½ teaspoon salt or Vege-Sal

½ teaspoon ground black pepper

½ cup (120 ml) chicken broth

YIELD: 6 servings

493 calories; 43 g fat; 25 g protein; 2 g carbohydrate; trace dietary fiber per serving

SPARERIBS *ADOBADO*

Spareribs are scrumptious, and a cheap, fatty cut that's perfect for us. But sugary barbecue sauce is out, so what to do? I love these, and since they're roasted in the oven, you can have them in January without tending the grill in the snow. They do take time though, so make them on a day when you're puttering around the house.

Preheat oven to 325ºF (170ºC, or gas mark 3).

Crush 2 cloves of the garlic, and stir into 1 tablespoon (15 ml) of the olive oil. Let it sit for 10 minutes. Then use clean hands to rub this mixture all over the ribs, coating both sides. Put 'em in a roasting pan.

In a small dish, stir together the seasonings. Remove 1 tablespoon (7 g) of the mixture to a small bowl, and reserve.

Sprinkle the ribs all over with the seasoning mixture that you didn't reserve in the bowl. Cover all sides. Put the ribs in to roast, and set your timer for 25 minutes (a few minutes one way or another won't matter).

While the ribs are roasting, crush the last clove of garlic and add to the reserved spice mixture with the chicken broth and the remaining 3 tablespoons (15 ml) olive oil.

Stir to combine. This is your mopping sauce.

When the timer goes off, baste your ribs with the mopping sauce, turning them over as you do so. Stick 'em back in the oven, and set the timer for another 20 minutes.

Repeat for a good 1½ to 2 hours; you want your ribs sizzling and brown all over and tender when you pierce them with a fork. Cut into individual ribs to serve.

SLOW-COOKER PORK CHILI

Try this when you want to have people over after the kids' soccer game. Toss a couple of bags of coleslaw mix with Coleslaw Dressing (page 73) for a cool contrasting accompaniment.

Heat the olive oil in your big, heavy skillet, and brown the pork cubes all over. Dump 'em in the slow cooker.

Stir in the tomatoes, onion, pepper, chili powder, and garlic . Cover and cook on low for 6 to 8 hours. Serve with sour cream and shredded Monterey Jack, if you like, but it's darned good as is.

1 tablespoon (15 ml) olive oil

2½ pounds (1.1 kg) boneless pork loin, cut into 1-inch (2.5 cm) cubes

1 can (14½ ounces, or 410 g) diced tomatoes with green chiles

¼ cup (40 g) chopped onion

¼ cup (38 g) diced green bell pepper

1 tablespoon (7.5 g) chili powder

1 clove garlic, crushed

Sour cream (optional)

Shredded Monterey Jack cheese (optional)

YIELD: 8 servings
189 calories; 8 g fat; 25 g protein; 3 g carbohydrate; 1 g dietary fiber per serving

MEDITERRANEAN LAMB BURGERS

This is about as upscale as a cheeseburger can get. My husband, who generally prefers beef to lamb, thought these were great.

Preheat your electric tabletop grill; I set mine to 350°F (180°C).

Chop your onion, and if your sun-dried tomatoes are in halves rather than prechopped, chop them up, too. Heck, even if they're prechopped, chop them a little more. Throw these things in a mixing bowl.

Add the ground lamb, pesto, garlic, salt, and pepper. Use clean hands to squish it all together until it's well mixed. Form into 3 patties and throw them on the grill. Set a timer for 5 minutes.

While the burgers are cooking, toast your pine nuts in a dry skillet until they're touched with gold.

When your burgers are done, plate them, crumble an ounce (28 g) of chèvre over each one, sprinkle with pine nuts, and then serve.

¼ medium onion

2 tablespoons (7 g) chopped sun-dried tomatoes

1 pound (455 g) ground lamb

1 tablespoon (15 g) pesto sauce

1 tablespoon (10 g) chopped garlic

½ teaspoon salt or Vege-Sal

¼ teaspoon ground black pepper

2 tablespoons (18 g) pine nuts

3 ounces (85 g) chèvre (goat cheese)

YIELD: 3 servings
578 calories; 47 g fat; 33 g protein; 4 g carbohydrate; 1 g dietary fiber per serving

1 package (10 ounces, or 280 g) frozen chopped spinach, thawed and drained

¼ cup (40 g) minced onion

1 tablespoon (15 ml) lemon juice

1 teaspoon dried basil

¼ teaspoon salt or Vege-Sal

¼ teaspoon ground black pepper

1 egg

1 clove garlic, minced fine

1¼ pounds (570 g) ground lamb

½ cup (75 g) crumbled feta cheese

¼ cup (15 g) chopped sun-dried tomatoes

12 kalamata olives, pitted and chopped

YIELD: 6 servings

352 calories; 28 g fat; 20 g protein; 5 g carbohydrate; 2 g dietary fiber per serving

LAMB, FETA, AND SPINACH BURGERS

Once again, a recipe I wrote for the electric tabletop grill, and once again, you can do them in your skillet if you prefer. If you're doing that, make them closer to ½ inch (1 cm) thick—the grill squishes them down. These have 5 grams of carbs apiece, but they include your vegetables.

Make sure your spinach is well drained—I put mine in a strainer and then squeeze it with clean hands. Transfer it to a big bowl, and add the onion, lemon juice, basil, salt, pepper, egg, and garlic. Stir it all up until it's well blended.

Now add the lamb, feta, tomatoes, and olives. Use clean hands to mix everything until it's really well combined. Make 6 burgers, keeping them at least 1 inch (2.5 cm) thick. I like to refrigerate them for at least 20 to 30 minutes before cooking.

Preheat your electric tabletop grill. Slap the burgers on the grill, and give 'em 6 to 8 minutes, depending on how well done you want them. I find that the burgers at the back of the grill brown sooner than the burgers at the front; don't be afraid to remove the ones that are done and continue cooking the others to your desired doneness.

LAMB STEAKS WITH LEMON, OLIVES, AND CAPERS

This is as good a fast dinner as I've ever made. Throw in a green salad with vinaigrette, crumble in some feta, and you're living large.

1½ pounds (680 g) leg of lamb in steaks, ¾ inch (2 cm) thick

2 teaspoons olive oil

1 tablespoon (15 ml) lemon juice

¼ cup (25 g) chopped kalamata olives

2 teaspoons capers

1 clove garlic

Salt and ground black pepper, to taste

YIELD: 4 servings

343 calories; 26 g fat; 24 g protein; 1 g carbohydrate; trace dietary fiber per serving

Coat your large, heavy skillet with nonstick cooking spray and put it over medium-high heat. While it's heating, slash the edges of your lamb steaks to keep them from curling. When the skillet's hot, add the oil, and throw in the steaks. You want to sear them on both sides.

When your steaks are browned on both sides, add the lemon juice, olives, capers, and garlic around and over the steaks. Let the whole thing cook another minute or two, but don't overcook—the lamb should still be pink in the middle. Season the steaks with salt and pepper, carve them into 4 portions, and serve with all the yummy lemon-caper-olive mixture from the skillet scraped over them.

ROMAN LAMB STEAK

This marinade really complements the flavor of the lamb. And don't fear those anchovies. The results aren't fishy, just very tasty.

¾ pound (340 g) leg of lamb steaks, ½ inch (1 cm) thick

½ cup (30 g) chopped fresh parsley

1 tablespoon (15 ml) olive oil

1 tablespoon (15 ml) lemon juice

¼ teaspoon ground black pepper

⅛ teaspoon salt

2 anchovy fillets

1 clove garlic, crushed

YIELD: 2 servings

387 calories; 30 g fat; 26 g protein; 2 g carbohydrate; 1 g dietary fiber per serving

Put your lamb steak on a plate. Throw everything else in your food processor with the S-blade in place, and pulse to chop the parsley, anchovies, and garlic into a coarse paste. Smear half of the resulting mixture on one side of the steak, turn it, and smear the rest on the other side. Now let the steak sit for at least half an hour—a couple of hours is great.

After marinating, preheat your broiler and broil the lamb close to the heat (with the parsley mixture still all over it) for about 6 minutes per side—it should still be pink in the middle—and serve.

1 pound (455 g) boneless leg of lamb, cubed

¼ cup (60 ml) olive oil

¼ cup (60 ml) lemon juice

4 cloves garlic, minced fine

1 medium onion

Salt and ground black pepper, to taste

YIELD: 4 servings

290 calories; 20 g fat; 24 g protein; 5 g carbohydrate; 1 g dietary fiber per serving (The carb count is high, since you'll throw away some of the marinade. You can afford a small salad.)

MIDDLE EASTERN MARINATED LAMB KABOBS

Whether you call it shish kebab or souvlaki, this is just good. Serve with a romaine salad with vinaigrette—French Vinaigrette (page 72) would be fine—and a few olives, a little feta, or both.

Put your lamb cubes in a big resealable plastic bag. Mix together the olive oil, lemon juice, and garlic and pour over the lamb. Seal the bag, pressing out the air as you go. Turn the bag once or twice to coat, and throw it in the fridge for several hours.

If you plan to use bamboo skewers, put them in water to soak about 30 minutes before cooking time.

Okay, time to decide if you're cooking these under the broiler or outside on your barbecue grill. If you want to cook them over charcoal—certainly a terrific way to go—get your fire going a good 30 minutes before you want to cook.

When dinner rolls around, cut your onion into hunks, and separate into individual layers. Pull out your lamb cubes, and pour off the marinade into a dish.

Thread the lamb cubes onto 4 skewers—I used metal ones. Alternate your lamb chunks with pieces of onion. Keep it compact, with stuff touching, not strung out. When the skewers are full, and all the lamb and onion is used up, sprinkle your kabobs with a little salt and pepper.

Now grill or broil, basting occasionally with the reserved marinade, for 8 to 10 minutes, or until done to your liking—I prefer my lamb to still be a bit pink in the middle. Stop basting with 3 to 4 minutes to go, to make sure any of the raw meat germs in the marinade get killed. Serve 1 skewer per customer.

5 scallions, divided

¼ cup (10 g) fresh basil leaves

1 pound (455 g) ground pork

1 tablespoon (15 ml) fish sauce (*nam pla* or *nuoc mam*)

1 tablespoon (15 g) chili garlic sauce (sometimes called *sambal oelek*)

1 tablespoon (1.5 g) Splenda, or the equivalent in liquid Splenda

2 teaspoons chopped garlic

1 teaspoon salt

1 teaspoon ground black pepper

⅓ cup (75 g) mayonnaise

1 tablespoon (15 g) chili garlic sauce

YIELD: 3 servings
597 calories; 5 g fat; 2 g protein; 5 g carbohydrate; 1 g dietary fiber per serving

BANH MI BURGERS

I saw a recipe for a Vietnamese meatball sandwich and thought, "I could make that into burgers." So I did. These are good with Asian Ginger Slaw (page 75), but plenty tasty on their own.

Preheat an electric tabletop grill. If you can choose temperature settings on yours, use 350°F (180°C).

Cut the root and any limp greens off the scallions, whack them into a few pieces, and throw three of them into your food processor with the S-blade in place. (Reserve the other two.) Throw in the basil, too. Pulse until they're finely chopped together.

Now add the pork, fish sauce, chili garlic sauce, Splenda, garlic, salt, and pepper to the processor and run it until everything is well blended.

Form the pork mixture into 3 patties and put them on the grill. Set a timer for 6 to 8 minutes.

Quickly wash out your food processor and reassemble with the S-blade in place. Put the remaining 2 scallions in there and pulse to chop. Now add the mayonnaise and chili sauce and run to blend.

When the burgers are done, serve with the sauce.

CHAPTER 12
Main Dish Salads

Putting this chapter together has been eye-opening. I have long thought main-dish salads to be one of the tastiest and most nutritious ways to eat low carb, yet I found that the vast majority of my main-dish salad recipes have more than 5 grams of total carbs. These are the ones that don't.

We're starting with a couple of versions of good old tuna salad, then egg salad. In case you've only ever had these as sandwich fillings, I'd like to tell you about a stunning new technological development that lets you get food from your plate to your mouth without the use of an edible napkin: It's called the fork. Use it!

2 big ribs celery or 3 smaller ones

½ green bell pepper

¼ medium sweet red onion

1 can (5 ounces, or 142 g) tuna packed in olive oil

⅓ cup (75 g) mayonnaise

2 tablespoons (30 g) minced sugar-free bread-and-butter pickles

---

YIELD: 2 servings
424 calories; 37 g fat; 22 g protein; 5 g carbohydrate; 2 g dietary fiber per serving

DANA'S TUNA SALAD

This is my lunchtime standby. With so many vegetables, this really is a tuna *salad*. Look for sugar-free bread-and-butter pickles alongside the regular pickles in your grocery store.

Dice up the vegetables—I like them fairly chunky, so I get lots of crunchy texture. This comes to 1½ to 2 cups of veggies! Then add the tuna, mayonnaise, and pickles, and mix it up. I've been known to eat this straight out of the mixing bowl. (Hey, I'm home alone at lunchtime. I'm allowed to eat out of the mixing bowl.)

1 can (5 ounces, or 142 g) tuna packed in olive oil

2 ribs celery

⅓ cup (55 g) diced sweet red onion

⅓ cup (20 g) chopped fresh parsley

1 tablespoon (9 g) capers

1 tablespoon (15 ml) lemon juice

1 tablespoon (14 g) mayonnaise

YIELD: 2 servings
212 calories; 12 g fat; 22 g protein; 5 g carbohydrate; 2 g dietary fiber per serving

TUNA SALAD WITH LEMON AND CAPERS

I've always loved the bright, sunny flavors of lemon and capers in *piccata*-style dishes. This is my way of adding those Mediterranean flavors to tuna salad.

Just drain your tuna lightly—you want some of the olive oil in the salad—and dice your celery. Add to a mixing bowl with everything else, and combine lightly.

4 hard-boiled eggs

1 rib celery, diced

4 scallions, sliced, including the crisp part of the green

5 green olives, pitted and chopped

⅓ cup (75 g) mayonnaise

Salt and ground black pepper, to taste

YIELD: 2 servings

443 calories; 43 g fat; 14 g protein; 5 g carbohydrate; 1 g dietary fiber per serving

JANE'S EGG SALAD

Jane was my mother, and she liked olives in her egg salad. Who am I to argue about something like that? It's really good.

Your basic egg salad procedure: Peel and coarsely chop your eggs, and cut up your veggies. Assemble everything in a mixing bowl, then stir it up gently, to preserve some hunks of yolk, till everything is evenly distributed. Season with salt and pepper to taste, and you're done.

1½ cups (210 g) diced leftover cooked chicken

¼ cup (28 g) chopped pecans

⅓ cup (75 g) mayonnaise

2 big ribs celery, diced

¼ medium sweet red onion, diced

Salt, to taste

YIELD: 2 servings

640 calories; 60 g fat; 24 g protein; 5 g carbohydrate; 2 g dietary fiber per serving

CHICKEN-PECAN SALAD

A good reason to cook an extra couple of pieces of chicken every time you're roasting some. This will keep you full for hours and hours.

Toss all ingredients together, salting to taste. That's it!

6 ounces (170 g) boneless, skinless chicken breast

3 cups (165 g) torn romaine lettuce

2 tablespoons (28 g) Caesar dressing, homemade or bottled

2 tablespoons (10 g) Parmesan cheese—fresh, in thin slivers, is nicest, but you can use the grated stuff if you like

---

YIELD: 1 serving

402 calories; 22 g fat; 44 g protein; 5 g carbohydrate; 2 g dietary fiber per serving

---

YIELD: 1 serving

317 calories; 19 g fat; 30 g protein; 5 g carbohydrate; 2 g dietary fiber per serving

CHICKEN CAESAR SALAD

This salad is a snap. (By the way, a chicken Caesar, hold the croutons, is a pretty safe choice at restaurants.) If you miss the crunch, try this: Use Parmesan with no additives—that part is important—and spread it on a microwavable plate you've coated with nonstick spray. Microwave it for a minute, then let it cool into a crunchy disk, and crumble it into the salad.

Start your chicken breast grilling; I do mine on an electric tabletop grill for about 5 minutes, but you could sauté it if you prefer.

Meanwhile, assemble your lettuce, pour the dressing over it, and toss well. Pile it on your serving plate.

When the chicken breast is done, slice it into thin strips, and pile it on top of the lettuce. Scatter the Parmesan over it, and dig in.

VARIATION: Shrimp Caesar Salad

Tired of chicken Caesar salads? Try this! With precooked shrimp, it's even quicker and easier. Just substitute 10 to 12 good-size cooked shrimp for the chicken breast. Frozen, precooked, peeled shrimp thaw quickly, especially if you put them in a resealable plastic bag and put them in warm tap water for a few minutes.

1 package (8 oz or 225 g) tofu shirataki, fettuccine width

3 tablespoons (20 g) slivered almonds

1½ teaspoons coconut oil

2 tablespoons (28 g) mayonnaise

1 tablespoon (16 g) almond butter

2 teaspoons soy sauce

½ teaspoon grated fresh ginger root

6 drops Sriracha

½ cup (70 g) cooked chicken

2 scallions

YIELD: 2 servings

298 calories; 26 g fat; 15 g protein; 5 g carbohydrate; 2 g dietary fiber per serving

CHICKEN-ALMOND NOODLE SALAD

Roughly a million years ago, when I was working at Chicago School of Massage Therapy, I used to walk out to a local health food store and—being sure that whole grains were good for me—buy a chicken, almond, and whole wheat pasta salad for lunch. It's been years, and I don't know how close this comes, but it's reminiscent of that salad. Darned good in its own right, anyway.

I used leftover roasted chicken for this—I always roast extra, for just such purposes. But if you have no cold chicken in the house, you could quickly cook a boneless, skinless breast.

Snip open the packet of tofu shirataki, and pour into a strainer in the sink. Rinse well, and use your kitchen shears to snip across them a couple of times, as they're so long. If you want, you can put them to soak in a bowl of fresh water, but I didn't bother.

Put the shirataki in a microwavable bowl, and nuke them on high for 2 minutes. Drain again, and repeat with another 2 minutes and another draining. Let them cool while you do the rest.

In a small, heavy skillet over medium-low heat, start your almonds sautéing in your coconut oil.

Measure your mayonnaise, almond butter, soy sauce, ginger root, and Sriracha into a smallish dish, and stir together. This is your dressing.

Go back and stir your almonds! In fact, stir 'em once in between measuring the dressing ingredients. You don't want them to burn. When they're just getting golden, take them off the heat.

Cut your chicken into ½-inch (1 cm) cubes. Thinly slice your scallions, including the crisp part of the green.

Okay, time to assemble your salad. Dump the shirataki into a mixing bowl. Add the chicken, scallions, toasted almonds, and then the dressing. Stir it all up, and you're done!

½ head cauliflower

2 cups (280 g) diced cooked turkey

1 heart romaine lettuce, cut crosswise in ½-inch (1 cm) strips—about 4 cups (220 g) lettuce

1 large tomato, diced

½ cup (115 g) mayonnaise

2 tablespoons (28 ml) cider vinegar

2 tablespoons (28 ml) lemon juice

1 teaspoon spicy brown mustard

10 slices bacon, cooked crisp

Salt and ground black pepper, to taste

YIELD: 6 servings
326 calories; 26 g fat; 21 g protein; 5 g carbohydrate; 2 g dietary fiber per serving

CLUB SANDWICH SALAD

All the flavors you loved in a club sandwich in a filling salad. I used deli turkey, and had the guys at the deli slice it ½ inch (1 cm) thick, which made for nice cubes. But how great a Thanksgiving-weekend lunch would this make?

Trim the leaves and the very bottom of the stem off your half head of cauliflower, whack it into chunks, and run it through the shredding blade of your food processor. Put the resulting "cauli-rice" into a microwavable casserole dish with a lid, add a couple of tablespoons (30 ml) of water, and nuke on high for 6 minutes.

In the meantime, throw your turkey, lettuce, and tomato in a big salad bowl.

When your microwave beeps, pull out your cauli-rice and uncover it to stop the cooking. Let it cool a few minutes, so it won't cook your lettuce and tomatoes! It will cool faster if you drain it, and stir it now and then.

Measure and whisk together your mayonnaise, vinegar, lemon juice, and mustard.

Use your kitchen shears to snip the bacon into the salad, cutting it every ¼ inch (6 mm) or so. Now add the cauli-rice, pour on the dressing, season with salt and pepper to taste, toss well, and serve.

1½ cups (210 g) cooked chicken, diced

1 large rib celery, diced

½ green bell pepper, diced

¼ medium sweet red onion, diced

3 tablespoons (42 g) mayonnaise

3 tablespoons (42 g) sour cream

1 teaspoon dried dill weed

Salt, to taste

YIELD: 2 servings
576 calories; 48 g fat; 33 g protein; 5 g carbohydrate; 1 g dietary fiber per serving

DILLED CHICKEN SALAD

Yummy, creamy, and rich. This is wonderful when made with leftover turkey, too.

Combine the chicken, celery, green pepper, and onion in a bowl.

In a separate bowl, mix together the mayonnaise, sour cream, and dill. Pour the mixture over the chicken and veggies, toss, add salt to taste, and serve.

½ head cauliflower

1 cup (100 g) diced celery

½ red bell pepper, diced

⅓ cup (55 g) diced red onion

¼ cup (60 g) diced green chiles

2 cups (280 g) diced cooked chicken

4 ounces (115 g) Monterey Jack cheese, cut into ¼-inch (6 mm) cubes

⅓ cup (75 g) mayonnaise

1 tablespoon (15 ml) white vinegar

1½ teaspoons lime juice

1 teaspoon chili powder

½ teaspoon ground cumin

½ teaspoon dried oregano

2 ounces (55 g) sliced black olives, drained

YIELD: 5 servings

418 calories; 34 g fat; 23 g protein; 5 g carbohydrate; 2 g dietary fiber per serving

CHICKEN-CHILI-CHEESE SALAD

You got your chicken, you got your vegetables, you got your cheese. Pretty nutritious, you think? All that, and it tastes good, too. Feel free to make this with leftover turkey or ham, if you prefer. Or, for that matter, with canned chunk chicken, should you not have any cold cooked chicken in the house.

First, chop your cauliflower into 1½-inch (3.8 cm) chunks. Throw it in a microwavable casserole dish with a lid, add a couple of tablespoons (30 ml) of water, cover, and nuke it on high for 7 minutes.

While that's cooking, assemble your other vegetables, chicken, and cheese in a big mixing bowl.

As soon as the microwave beeps, pull out your cauliflower, uncover it, and drain it. Let it sit and cool for a few minutes. You don't want it to melt your cheese. The cauliflower will cool faster if you stir it now and then.

While you're waiting for the cauliflower to cool, measure your mayonnaise, vinegar, lime juice, chili powder, cumin, and oregano. Stir it all together.

Okay, cauliflower cooled a bit? Dump it in with the chicken, cheese, and veggies, and stir everything 'round. Dump in the olives, pour on the dressing, and toss to coat. You can eat this right away, if you'd like, or chill it for a few hours.

6 cups (510 g) fresh broccoli florets

1½ cups (173 g) shredded Cheddar cheese

⅓ cup (55 g) chopped onion

1½ cups (335 g) mayonnaise

½ to ¾ cup (12 to 18 g) Splenda*

3 tablespoons (45 ml) red wine vinegar or cider vinegar

12 slices bacon, cooked and crumbled

---

*Alternative Sweeteners

½ to ¾ cup (24 to 36 g) Stevia in the Raw

½ to ¾ teaspoon liquid stevia (plain)

¼ to ⅓ teaspoon EZ-Sweetz Family Size

12 to 18 drops EZ-Sweetz Travel Size

YIELD: 8 servings

455 calories; 47 g fat; 10 g protein; 4 g carbohydrate; 2 g dietary fiber per serving

CHEDDAR-BROCCOLI SALAD

Our tester called this recipe that reader Eleanor Monfett donated for *500 More Low-Carb Recipes* "great stuff." It's not a traditional main-dish salad, but it has so much cheese and bacon that it sure can serve as one.

In a large bowl, combine the broccoli, cheese and onion. Combine the mayonnaise, Splenda, and vinegar; pour over the broccoli mixture and toss to coat. Refrigerate for at least 4 hours. Just before serving, stir in the bacon.

If you prefer, you can lightly steam the broccoli, then cool before adding the other ingredients. But don't go beyond tender-crisp.

6 ounces (170 g) sirloin steak, 1 inch (2.5 cm) thick

1 cup torn romaine lettuce

1 tablespoon (15 ml) vinaigrette—French Vinaigrette (page 72) or Italian Vinaigrette (page 72) would be good

2 tablespoons (16 g) minced red onion

2 tablespoons (16 g) crumbled blue cheese

¼ large tomato, cut into wedges

YIELD: 1 serving

496 calories; 36 g fat; 36 g protein; 5 g carbohydrate; 2 g dietary fiber per serving

SIRLOIN SALAD

The original version of this salad had too many vegetables for the HEAL Protocol. I adapted it, and it's still wonderful. It's easy to double or even triple—just grill a bigger steak. For that matter, in the unlikely event you should have leftover steak, this is a great way to turn it into a fresh meal.

Preheat your grill or broiler and cook the steak to your liking—I'd go with medium-rare.

Meanwhile, toss the lettuce with the vinaigrette and arrange it on a plate.

When your steak is done, slice it medium-thin across the grain, and arrange it on the bed of lettuce. Scatter the onion and cheese over it, arrange the tomato wedges around it, and it's done.

CHAPTER 13
Soups

Soup is wonderful stuff—comforting, warming, filling. Sadly, most packaged soups include carb-laden ingredients, including noodles, rice, potatoes, barley, and cornstarch. Even generous quantities of the more carb-heavy vegetables can send soup past our 5-gram limit. Fortunately, homemade soup is not only easy but far tastier than the canned, powdered, or frozen types.

For super-nutritious soup, use homemade bone broth. This is easy and virtually free. Here's how I do it: I save all the bones from roast chicken, rotisserie chicken, chicken wings—all of them—in a plastic grocery sack in my freezer. No matter how clean the bones are picked, they still are great for broth. I also add onion, carrot, and celery trimmings, going easy on celery leaves, which can turn bitter. When I have enough to fill my big slow cooker, I dump them in, still frozen, and cover them with water. I add a tablespoon or two (15 to 28 ml) of cider or wine vinegar and a teaspoon of salt, cover the slow cooker, and let it cook for a good 24 hours. Once cooled and strained, it's ready to be used or frozen. A stash of good broth in the freezer is culinary gold.

However, good packaged broth or stock is worth keeping on hand. You'll want to read the labels. I like Kitchen Basics brand; it contains no junk, though it has a touch of honey. Between that and the vegetables used, it comes to 1 gram of carbohydrate per serving. Kitchen Basics comes in chicken, beef, and seafood varieties, which are all useful for us.

1 large or 2 small avocados, very ripe

1 quart (950 ml) hot chicken broth

YIELD: 6 appetizer-size servings
80 calories; 6 g fat; 4 g protein; 3 g carbohydrate; 1 g dietary fiber per serving

CALIFORNIA SOUP

A quick and elegant first course. If you like curry, try adding ½ to 1 teaspoon or so of curry powder that you've cooked for just a minute or two in a tablespoon (14 g) of butter.

Pit and peel the avocado, and cut it into big chunks. Purée in the blender with the broth (use caution when blending hot liquids) until very smooth, and serve.

1 quart (950 ml) chicken broth, divided

½ teaspoon guar or xanthan

1 cup (100 g) minced black olives (you can buy cans of minced black olives)

1 cup (235 ml) heavy cream

¼ cup (60 ml) dry sherry

Salt or Vege-Sal and ground black pepper, to taste

YIELD: 6 appetizer-size servings
189 calories; 17 g fat; 2 g protein; 3 g carbohydrate; 1 g dietary fiber per serving

OLIVE SOUP

Olives are so good for you that you should be eating more of them! This makes a fine first course.

Put ½ cup (120 ml) of the chicken broth in the blender with the guar and blend for a few seconds. Pour into a saucepan and add the remaining 3½ cups (830 ml) broth and the olives.

Heat until simmering, then whisk in the cream. Bring back to a simmer, stir in the sherry, and season with salt and pepper to taste.

1 quart (950 ml) chicken broth, divided

¼ teaspoon guar or xanthan (optional)

1 tablespoon (15 ml) soy sauce

1 tablespoon (15 ml) rice vinegar

½ teaspoon grated fresh ginger root

1 scallion, sliced

2 eggs

YIELD: 4 appetizer-size servings
75 calories; 4 g fat; 8 g protein; 2 g carbohydrate; trace dietary fiber per serving

EGG DROP SOUP

This soup is quick and easy, but filling, and it can practically save your life when you've got a cold. You don't have to use the guar, but it gives the broth the same rich quality that cornstarch-thickened Chinese broths have.

Put 1 cup (240 ml) or so of the chicken broth in your blender, turn it on low, and add the guar (if using). Let it blend for a second, then put it in a large saucepan with the remaining 3 cups (710 ml) broth. (If you're not using guar or xanthan, just put all the broth directly in a saucepan.)

Add the soy sauce, rice vinegar, ginger, and scallion. Over medium-high heat, bring to a simmer and cook for 5 minutes or so to let the flavors blend.

Beat your eggs in a glass measuring cup or small pitcher—something with a pouring lip. Use a fork to stir the surface of the soup in a slow circle and pour in about one-quarter of the eggs, stirring as they cook and turn into shreds (which will happen almost instantaneously). Repeat 3 more times, using up all the egg. That's it.

2 quarts (2 L) chicken broth

2 teaspoons grated fresh ginger root

1 pound (455 g) asparagus

2 eggs

1½ tablespoons (22 ml) dry sherry

1 tablespoon (15 ml) soy sauce

2 teaspoons dark sesame oil

12 ounces (340 g) lump crabmeat, fresh or canned

YIELD: 4 servings
237 calories; 8 g fat; 31 g protein; 5 g carbohydrate; 1 g dietary fiber per serving

CRAB AND ASPARAGUS SOUP

If you love egg drop soup, this is a fantastic twist on the original. Our tester Julie's son Austin calls it "the second best Dana recipe I've ever had!" (His favorite is the Roasted Asparagus on page 87.)

In a large, heavy saucepan, start the broth warming over medium heat. Stir in the ginger root.

Now snap the ends off of your asparagus where it wants to break naturally. Discard the ends, and slice the asparagus on the diagonal into ½-inch (1 cm) pieces. When the soup is simmering, add the asparagus to it. Let it simmer for about 3 minutes.

While that's happening, beat the eggs until blended in a glass measuring cup. When the asparagus is just barely tender-crisp, take a fork in one hand and the cup of beaten egg in the other. Pour a stream of egg onto the surface of the soup, then stir with the fork. Repeat. It should take 3 or 4 additions to stir in all the egg. Now you have lovely egg drops!

Stir in the sherry, soy sauce, and sesame oil. Now add the crab, stir again, and cook for another 5 minutes or so before serving.

1 quart (950 ml) chicken broth, divided

2 eggs

½ cup (50 g) grated Parmesan cheese

½ teaspoon lemon juice

Pinch of ground nutmeg

½ teaspoon dried marjoram

YIELD: 4 appetizer-size servings
117 calories; 7 g fat; 12 g protein; 2 g carbohydrate; trace dietary fiber per serving

STRACCIATELLA

This is the Italian take on egg drop soup, and it's delightful. And it has the added nutrition of cheese!

Put ¼ cup (60 ml) of the broth into a glass measuring cup or small pitcher. Pour the rest into a large saucepan over medium heat.

Add the eggs to the broth in the measuring cup and beat with a fork. Then add the Parmesan, lemon juice, and nutmeg, and beat with a fork until well blended.

When the broth in the saucepan is simmering, stir it with a fork as you add small amounts of the egg-and-cheese mixture, until it's all stirred in. (Don't expect this to form long shreds like Chinese egg drop soup; because of the Parmesan, it makes small, fluffy particles instead.)

Add the marjoram, crushing it a bit between your fingers, and simmer the soup for another minute or so before serving.

8 ounces (225 g) mushrooms, sliced

¼ cup (40 g) chopped onion

2 tablespoons (28 g) butter

1 quart (950 ml) chicken broth

½ cup (120 ml) heavy cream

½ cup (115 g) sour cream

Salt and ground black pepper, to taste

Guar or xanthan (optional)

YIELD: 5 servings
217 calories; 19 g fat; 6 g protein; 5 g carbohydrate; 1 g dietary fiber per serving

CREAM OF MUSHROOM SOUP

If you've only ever thought of mushroom soup as gooey stuff that comes in cans and is used in casseroles, you need to try this! It has a rich, earthy flavor. Even my mushroom-phobic husband liked it.

In a big, heavy skillet, sauté the mushrooms and onion in the butter until the mushrooms soften and change color. Transfer them to your slow cooker. Add the broth. Cover the slow cooker, set it to low, and let it cook for 5 to 6 hours.

When the time's up, scoop out the vegetables with a slotted spoon and put them in your blender or food processor. Add enough broth to help them process easily and purée them finely. Pour the puréed vegetables back into the slow cooker, scraping out every last bit with a rubber scraper.

Now stir in the heavy cream and sour cream and season with salt and pepper to taste. Thicken a bit with guar or xanthan if you think it needs it. Serve immediately.

1½ quarts (1.5 L) chicken broth, divided

1 pound (455 g) boneless, skinless chicken breast

1 chipotle chile canned in adobo

1 Hass avocado

4 scallions, sliced

Salt and ground black pepper, to taste

¾ cup (85 g) shredded Monterey Jack cheese

YIELD: 6 servings
235 calories; 13 g fat; 26 g protein; 4 g carbohydrate; 2 g dietary fiber per serving

SOPA TLALPEÑO

This simple Mexican soup takes no more than 25 minutes!

Pour the chicken broth into a large, heavy-bottomed saucepan, reserving ½ cup (120 ml), and place it over medium-high heat. While it's heating, cut your chicken breast into thin strips or small cubes, then add to the broth. Let the whole thing simmer for 10 to 15 minutes, or until the chicken is cooked through.

Put the reserved chicken broth in your blender with the chipotle and blend until the chipotle is puréed. Pour this mixture into the soup and stir.

Split the avocado in half, remove the seed, peel it, and cut it into ½-inch (1 cm) chunks. Add to the soup, along with the scallions, and salt and pepper to taste.

Ladle the soup into bowls and top each serving with shredded cheese.

1½ tablespoons (22 g) butter

¼ cup (40 g) finely minced onion

¼ cup (30 g) finely minced celery

2 cups (475 ml) heavy cream

1 can (14 ounces, or 390 g) salmon, drained

½ teaspoon dried thyme

YIELD: 4 servings
594 calories; 54 g fat; 23 g protein; 5 g carbohydrate; trace dietary fiber per serving

CREAM OF SALMON SOUP

My friend Chris, who has been coming to clean my house for a couple of decades now, sampled this soup and pronounced it the best she'd ever had. And it's so easy!

In a heavy saucepan, melt the butter over medium-low heat and add the onion and celery. Sauté the vegetables for a few minutes, until the onion starts turning translucent.

Meanwhile, pour the cream into a glass 2-cup (475 ml) measure, or any other microwavable container similar in size with a pouring spout. Place it in the microwave and heat it at 50 percent power for 3 to 4 minutes. (This just cuts the time needed to heat the cream through—you can skip this step and simply heat the soup on the stove top for a little longer, if you prefer.)

Pour the cream into the saucepan and add the salmon and thyme. Break up the salmon as you stir the soup—I found my whisk to be ideal for breaking the salmon into fine pieces. Heat until simmering, and serve.

CHINESE-STYLE TUNA SOUP

Quick, easy, and good. I admit that olive oil isn't Chinese, but it's better for you than the soybean oil typically found in cans of tuna.

1 quart (950 ml) chicken broth

2 teaspoons soy sauce

1 teaspoon grated fresh ginger root

2 eggs

1 can (6 ounces, or 170 g) tuna packed in olive oil

1½ cups (84 g) chopped fresh spinach

2 scallions, sliced thin

In a big saucepan, combine the chicken broth with the soy sauce and ginger. Put it over medium-high heat, and bring it to a boil, then turn the heat down till the broth is just simmering.

While the broth is heating, break the eggs into a little glass measuring cup, or another container with a pouring lip. Beat 'em up with a fork. When your soup is simmering, pour one-third of the egg into the soup, wait just 1 or 2 seconds, then stir with a fork, drawing out the egg into strands. Repeat with the rest of the egg, in 2 or 3 more additions.

When you're done adding the egg, add the tuna and spinach. Heat through and serve with scallions on top.

YIELD: 3 servings

216 calories; 9 g fat; 27 g protein; 3 g carbohydrate; 1 g dietary fiber per serving

TAVERN SOUP

Cheese soup with beer! Don't worry about the kids—the alcohol cooks off. Michelob Ultra, Miller Light, or Milwaukee's Best Light are the lowest in carbs.

1½ quarts (1.5 L) chicken broth

¼ cup (30 g) finely diced celery

¼ cup (30 g) finely diced green bell pepper

¼ cup (30 g) shredded carrot

¼ cup (15 g) chopped fresh parsley

½ teaspoon ground black pepper

1 pound (455 g) sharp Cheddar cheese, shredded

12 ounces (355 ml) light beer

½ teaspoon salt or Vege-Sal

¼ teaspoon hot pepper sauce

Guar or xanthan, as needed

Combine the broth, celery, green pepper, carrot, parsley, and black pepper in your slow cooker. Cover the pot, set the slow cooker to low, and let it cook for 6 to 8 hours (longer won't hurt).

When the time's up, either use a handheld blender to purée the vegetables right there in the slow cooker or scoop them out with a slotted spoon, purée them in your blender, and return them to the slow cooker.

Now whisk in the cheese a little at a time, until it's all melted in. Add the beer, salt, and hot pepper sauce, and stir until the foaming stops. Use guar as needed to thicken your soup until it's about the texture of heavy cream. Re-cover the pot, turn the slow cooker to high, and let it cook for another 20 minutes before serving.

YIELD: 8 servings

274 calories; 20 g fat; 18 g protein; 3 g carbohydrate; trace dietary fiber per serving

3 tablespoons (42 g) butter

½ cup (80 g) chopped onion

½ cup (50 g) chopped celery

1 medium carrot, grated

4 ounces (115 g) ham

4 cans (14½ ounces, or 441 g, each) green beans

½ teaspoon dried thyme

2 bay leaves

2 pinches of cayenne

Salt and ground black pepper, to taste

YIELD: 5 servings
120 calories; 9 g fat; 5 g protein; 5 g carbohydrate; 1 g dietary fiber per serving

NOT PEA SOUP

One of the few carb-heavy foods I miss is split pea soup, so I came up with this. It's not exactly like split pea soup, but it's similar, and it satisfied my craving. It's also quick and easy to make.

In a heavy saucepan, melt the butter and start sautéing the onion, celery, and carrot over medium heat.

While that's happening, put your ham in your food processor with the S-blade in place, and pulse until it's chopped medium-fine. Scrape this out of the food processor and into the saucepan with the veggies. Give everything a stir while you're there.

Return the processor bowl to its base, and put the S-blade back in. Dump in the green beans, liquid and all, and run the processor until the beans are pureed quite smooth.

Go back and look at your sautéing vegetables; when they are soft, add the garlic. Sauté it with the vegetables for just a minute.

Now dump in your green bean puree, and stir everything together. Add the thyme, bay leaves, and cayenne, and stir them in. Turn the heat to low, and bring the soup to a simmer. Let it cook for 15 minutes or so.

Season with salt and pepper to taste, remove the bay leaves, and pour into mugs.

CHAPTER 14
Sauces and Seasonings

Sauces, condiments, spice rubs, and sprinkle-on seasonings create great variety in our diets. Unfortunately, a dismaying number of commercially available flavorings are sources of sugar, often in meaningful quantities. When you're limited to 20 grams of carbohydrate per day, "spending" 8 grams on a couple of tablespoons (34 g) of ketchup is extravagant—and barbecue sauce runs 10 to 15 grams! You need alternatives.

Fortunately, Heinz, the undisputed king of ketchup, makes Reduced Sugar Ketchup (they can't call it "sugar free" because tomatoes have sugar in them) running just 1 gram of carbohydrate per tablespoon (15 g). I've been known to make my own ketchup, but Heinz Reduced Sugar Ketchup tastes just like the regular stuff, and has become a staple in my kitchen.

Here is a broad selection of sauces and seasonings that will add variety to your already luxurious meals.

2/3 cup (160 ml) heavy cream

1/4 cup (50 g) whipped cream cheese

5 ounces (140 g) Cheddar cheese, shredded

1 teaspoon horseradish mustard (optional)

YIELD: 4 servings or 1 cup (235 g)

316 calories; 30 g fat; 10 g protein; 2 g carbohydrate; trace dietary fiber per serving

CHEESE SAUCE

This is tremendous over broccoli or cauliflower. But its highest use is over tofu shirataki for mac and cheese.

In a saucepan over the lowest heat, heat the cream and cream cheese together, whisking until they're combined. Whisk in the Cheddar a little at a time, letting each addition melt before adding more.

Whisk in the horseradish mustard, if using, and you're done.

1/3 cup (80 g) Heinz Reduced Sugar Ketchup

1 tablespoon (15 ml) Tabasco sauce (or Frank's RedHot or Louisiana brand), or to taste

1 tablespoon (15 ml) lemon juice

1 tablespoon (15 g) prepared horseradish

YIELD: 6 servings or 1/2 cup (120 g)

2 calories; trace fat; trace protein; 1 g carbohydrate; trace dietary fiber per serving

COCKTAIL SAUCE

This couldn't be easier, and it turns precooked shrimp from the grocery store into a great light meal. You could even get fancy and serve it on a bed of shredded iceberg lettuce, for a classic shrimp cocktail. Great with other kinds of seafood, too.

Just mix everything together. Done!

8 ounces (230 g) blue cheese, crumbled

¾ cup (165 g) softened butter

1 or 2 cloves garlic, crushed

1 tablespoon (11 g) spicy brown mustard

2 or 3 drops Tabasco sauce

YIELD: 8 servings

255 calories; 26 g fat; 6 g protein; 1 g carbohydrate; trace dietary fiber per serving

BLUE CHEESE STEAK BUTTER

This is one of those recipes that would have horrified me back in my low-fat days—and it's sooooo good! If you don't have a food processor, you can make this without one, it will just take some vigorous mixing. The "proper" way to serve steak butter is to spoon it onto foil or waxed paper and form it into a nice roll, which you then chill and cut into tidy slices to melt on steak. If you have that sort of patience, more power to you. I'll go with a bowl and spoon.

Just plunk all this stuff in your food processor and run it until it's well blended and smooth. Now taste it—do you want a bit more mustard? A little salt and pepper? A dash more Tabasco?

When it's so good you want to cry, put it in a pretty dish and chill it. Then drop a good, rounded tablespoonful over each serving of freshly grilled or broiled steak. You'll get roughly 8 rounded tablespoons out of this batch; each will have 1 gram of carbohydrate.

By the way, if you have steak-loving people on your holiday gift list—and hey, who doesn't?—a log of this steak butter wrapped in foil makes a nice present.

4 slices bacon

½ cup (112 g) butter

1 teaspoon spicy brown or Dijon mustard

YIELD: 4 servings

120 calories; 13 g fat; 1 g protein; trace carbohydrate; trace dietary fiber per serving

BACON BUTTER

Take that, low-fat pundits! This is great on steaks or burgers, but try it melted over fried eggs, too.

Lay your bacon on a microwave bacon rack or in a glass pie plate. Microwave on high for 4 to 5 minutes, or until crisp.

In the meantime, throw your butter in your food processor and add the mustard. Pulse until well combined.

By now your bacon is done. Pull it out of the microwave and use your kitchen shears to snip it into the food processor in little bits. Pulse the food processor to mix in the bacon. The more you pulse, the finer the bacon bits will be; go by your own preference.

3 cloves garlic

½ teaspoon salt

2 egg yolks

1 cup (235 ml) oil—I'd go with half virgin olive oil, half something blander—MCT oil, high-heat sunflower, or light olive oil

---

YIELD: 12 servings or 1½ cups (355 mg)

172 calories; 19 g fat; 1 g protein; trace carbohydrate; trace dietary fiber per serving

AIOLI

A garlicky riff on mayonnaise that's good on artichokes, asparagus, fish, chicken, or even topping crab cakes or salmon patties. To change it up, double the lemon juice and add a little grated lemon zest.

Put your garlic cloves and salt in your food processor, and run till the garlic is pulverized.

Add the egg yolks, and run till everything is well blended. While that's happening, you can measure your oil into a measuring cup with a pouring lip.

Now with the processor running, pour in the oil in a very thin stream, about the diameter of a pencil lead. When it's all in, it's done! Store in a lidded jar in the fridge.

½ cup (115 g) mayonnaise

2 packed tablespoons (7 g) chopped sun-dried tomatoes

2 packed tablespoons (5 g) chopped fresh basil

1 tablespoon (15 ml) lemon juice

1 teaspoon water

1 clove garlic, minced

YIELD: 12 servings or ¾ cup (175 g)

68 calories; 8 g fat; trace protein; 1 g carbohydrate; trace dietary fiber per serving

SUN-DRIED TOMATO AND BASIL MAYONNAISE

Intense sun-dried tomato flavor. Consider using this on grilled fish steaks or chicken.

Put everything in your food processor with the S blade in place. Now run the processor, stopping it every now and then to scrape down the sides with a rubber scraper to get things back into the path of the blade. You want the basil and tomatoes chopped up pretty finely, and you want the mayonnaise to have taken on a little pinky-brown color.

½ cup (115 g) mayonnaise

2 teaspoons soy sauce

1 teaspoon lemon juice

1 teaspoon wasabi paste

3 drops liquid stevia

YIELD: 8 servings or ½ cup (120 g)

100 calories; 12 g fat; trace protein; trace carbohydrate; trace dietary fiber per serving

¼ cup (60 g) erythritol*

2 tablespoons (14 g) paprika

1 tablespoon (15 g) celery salt

1 tablespoon (8 g) chili powder

1 tablespoon (9 g) garlic powder

1 tablespoon (7 g) onion powder

1 tablespoon (18 g) seasoned salt

2 teaspoons black pepper

1 teaspoon lemon pepper

1 teaspoon dry mustard

1 teaspoon dried sage

½ teaspoon cayenne

½ teaspoon dried thyme

---

*Alternative Sweeteners

¼ cup (6 g) Splenda

¼ cup (12 g) Stevia in the Raw

YIELD: 13 servings or a generous ¾ cup (175 g)

15 calories; trace fat; 1 g protein; 3 g carbohydrate; 1 g dietary fiber per serving

WASABI MAYONNAISE

Oh, my gosh, is this fabulous! Fabulous, fabulous, fabulous. On asparagus. On shrimp. On artichokes. On fingers. Just fabulous.

Just combine everything in a bowl, and whisk together well. Unbelievably good.

CLASSIC RUB

Sprinkle on pork or chicken before slow smoking for a true barbecue flavor. Good as a sprinkle-on seasoning at the table, too.

Just stir everything together. Store in a clean old spice shaker.

¼ cup (72 g) salt or Vege-Sal

3 tablespoons (21 g) ground cumin

3 tablespoons (27 g) garlic powder

2 tablespoons (12 g) ground black pepper

2 tablespoons (15 g) chili powder

2 tablespoons (3 g) Splenda or (6 g) Stevia in the Raw

1 tablespoon (15 g) erythritol

1 tablespoon (7 g) onion powder

2 teaspoons cocoa powder

YIELD: 16 servings or a generous 1 cup (235 g)

17 calories; trace fat; 1 g protein; 3 g carbohydrate; 1 g dietary fiber per serving

CHILI-COCOA RUB

I originally made this for steak. Then I tried it on pork and chicken and realized it was way too good to limit that way. Make this up, keep it in a shaker by the stove, and use it to improve all manner of things! It's the best rub I've come up with in a long time.

Stir everything together and store in a clean used spice shaker. Use on steaks, pork chops, burgers, ribs, you name it. It's so good!

½ cup (120 g) chive-and-onion cream cheese

2 tablespoons (28 ml) heavy cream

1 tablespoon (14 g) butter

1 clove garlic, crushed

2 tablespoons (10 g) grated Parmesan cheese

YIELD: 4 servings or about ¾ cup (175 g)

134 calories; 13 g fat; 2 g protein; 1 g carbohydrate; trace dietary fiber per serving

EASY ALFREDO SAUCE

Lovely over tofu shirataki—the fettuccine style, of course, for fettuccine Alfredo. But try it over broccoli or chicken, too. Or, for bonus points, broccoli, chicken, and tofu shirataki fettuccine!

In a small saucepan over low heat, combine the chive cream cheese, heavy cream, butter, and garlic. Whisk until you have a smooth sauce. Whisk in the Parmesan, and you're done.

¼ cup (6 g) Splenda, (12 g) Stevia in the Raw, or (60 g) erythritol

1 tablespoon (4 g) ground cinnamon

YIELD: 10 servings or about ⅓ cup (80 g)

4 calories; trace protein; 1 g carbohydrate; trace dietary fiber per serving

CINNAMON "SUGAR"

Maple syrup is out, but with this super-simple topping for pancakes, waffles, and the like, you'll never miss it.

Dead simple: Stir the two together. That's it.

½ cup (112 g) butter, softened

⅛ teaspoon maple extract

20 drops liquid stevia (English toffee)

YIELD: 8 servings or about ½ cup (112 g)

102 calories; 11 g fat; trace protein; trace carbohydrate; 0 g dietary fiber per serving

MAPLE BUTTER

A great alternative to sugar-free pancake syrup—all the maple flavor, none of the carbs. Great on pancakes and waffles, of course, but also wonderful for roasting turnips. I got the maple extract (Boyajian brand) through Amazon.com.

Just run everything through the food processor till it's combined. Store in an airtight container in the fridge.

1 tablespoon (14 g) butter

1 shallot, minced

¾ cup (180 ml) half-and-half

1 cup (120 g) crumbled
Gorgonzola cheese

YIELD: 4 servings

186 calories; 16 g fat; 7 g protein;
3 g carbohydrate; 1 g dietary fiber
per serving

GORGONZOLA SAUCE

This sinfully rich sauce turns a simple chicken breast into a gourmet meal. Also good tossed with shirataki noodles. Gorgonzola's mild blue cheese flavor is especially good here, but you could use any soft domestic blue cheese.

In a heavy saucepan, melt the butter over medium-low heat and start sautéing the minced shallot. When it's soft, add the half-and-half and the crumbled Gorgonzola. Turn the heat down to low and cook, stirring often, until the Gorgonzola is melted.

3 tablespoons (45 g) erythritol

1 tablespoon (15 ml) water

1 chipotle chile canned in adobo

1 clove garlic, crushed

6 drops liquid stevia (English
toffee)

6 drops maple extract

YIELD: 5 servings or about ¼ cup
(60 g)

1 calorie; trace fat; trace protein;
trace carbohydrate; trace dietary
fiber per serving

MAPLE-CHIPOTLE GLAZE

This is good for basting chicken or pork, but even better for basting salmon steaks!

Put everything in your food processor, and run it till the chipotle's minced fine.

1 cup (225 g) mayonnaise

1 chipotle chile canned in adobo

½ teaspoon ground cumin

1 clove garlic

YIELD: 16 servings or 1 cup (235 g)

99 calories; 12 g fat; trace protein; trace carbohydrate; trace dietary fiber per serving

CHIPOTLE MAYONNAISE

Good for dipping chicken or shrimp, even roasted asparagus. A dollop atop an omelet wouldn't go amiss, either.

Put everything in your food processor, and run till the chipotle and garlic are pulverized. That's it.

CHAPTER 15
Beverages

Of all the changes you can make to your diet, the most beneficial is quitting sugary beverages. Americans swill down a stunning quantity of sugar in the form of coffee drinks, energy drinks, sports drinks, sugared teas, and, of course, sodas you could high-dive into.

How much? According to the CDC, men are consuming on average 178 calories per day in sugary drinks. At 4 calories per gram, that's 44.5 grams, or about 3½ tablespoons—just under ¼ cup of sugar per day in beverages alone. Women are getting 103 calories of sugared beverages per day, or 25.75 grams, or about 2 tablespoons. That's a scary quantity of sugar—remember, you need only 1 teaspoon (4 grams) of sugar in your bloodstream at any time.

We're not going to tell you that diet soda is health food. But if you're a soda addict and have diabetes, and diet soda lets you make the shift to a low-carbohydrate diet, we say bring it on. If you're concerned about artificial sweeteners, there are now a couple of brands of natural sugar-free soda on the market, Zevia and Blue Sky Free, both sweetened with erythritol and stevia. If your local health food stores or supermarkets don't carry these, ask if they can order them—or better yet, suggest they stock them. With an item this heavy, ordering through a store rather than online can save you substantial shipping fees.

"Drink water!" the health pundits cry. Yes, water is great, but is it the only healthful beverage? Hah. Coffee and tea both contain beneficial antioxidants, as do herbal teas. Sparkling water is a great choice as well, and comes in a burgeoning variety of flavors. Read labels—there are clear sodas out there that are labeled "sparkling water" or "seltzer," but contain sugar or corn syrup. LaCroix, Polar, Canada Dry, Perrier, and Ice Mountain are all widely available. Kroger, the nation's biggest grocery-store chain, now has a house brand of seltzer in several flavors.

All the beverages in this chapter are sweetened. Do not assume from this that you should drink all sweetened beverages. I drink unsweetened tea, hot or iced depending on the weather, during the day, and switch to unsweetened sparkling water in the evenings. I find these unsweetened beverages far more refreshing than sweet ones. So, this chapter contains sweet drinks because you can figure out the unsweetened ones by yourself.

We'll start with a couple of coffee drinks that work as great grab-and-go breakfasts for the morning-meal averse.

1 cup (235 ml) hot brewed coffee

2 tablespoons (16 g) chocolate whey protein powder

1½ tablespoons (22 g) unsalted grass-fed butter

1½ tablespoons (21 g) coconut oil

¼ teaspoon liquid stevia (chocolate)

YIELD: 1 serving

452 calories; 40 g fat; 23 g protein; 5 g carbohydrate; 2 g dietary fiber per serving

POWER PACK MOCHA

With plenty of appetite-curbing ketogenic fats and more protein than 3 eggs, this cup of coffee will keep your energy high and your mind clear all morning long. It'll do great things for your willpower, too. Worried about greasy coffee? You'll be surprised how creamy this is.

Feel free to make this with vanilla stevia and vanilla whey protein instead of the chocolate. If you're a stevia hater, try it with 1 to 2 tablespoons (15 to 28 ml) sugar-free chocolate or vanilla coffee flavoring syrup. For that matter, you could also use sugar-fee caramel syrup.

Just assemble everything in your blender and run till the butter and coconut oil are worked in and the whole thing is frothy. Pour into a travel mug and run!

1 cup (235 ml) brewed coffee, chilled

½ cup (120 ml) unsweetened canned coconut milk

1 tablespoon (8 g) chocolate whey protein powder

¼ teaspoon liquid stevia (chocolate)*

*Alternative Sweeteners

¼ cup (60 ml) chocolate sugar-free coffee flavoring syrup

12 drops EZ-Sweetz Family Size

6 drops EZ-Sweetz Travel Size

(If using EZ-Sweetz, add a little chocolate extract.)

YIELD: 1 serving

282 calories; 25 g fat; 13 g protein; 5 g carbohydrate; trace dietary fiber per serving

MORNING MOCHA

Somewhere between iced coffee and chocolate milk, this combines protein, highly ketogenic fat, and caffeine in one get-out-the-door package. Make it the night before, pour it into a travel mug, and chill for a super-streamlined morning. A 13½-ounce (398 ml) can of coconut milk holds roughly a cup and a half (355 ml)—close enough for making a triple batch, for even easier mornings.

Just run everything through the blender, pour, and go.

¾ cup (175 ml) brewed coffee

2 tablespoons (28 ml) sugar-free chocolate coffee flavoring syrup

2 tablespoons (28 ml) heavy cream

Tiny pinch of ground cinnamon

YIELD: 1 serving

106 calories; 11 g fat; 1 g protein; 2 g carbohydrate; trace dietary fiber per serving

CAFÉ VIENNA

Coffee for chocolate lovers, or chocolate for coffee lovers. Either way, it's charming. To spiff this up for company, used whipped cream instead of the plain heavy cream.

Pour the coffee, stir in the chocolate syrup and heavy cream, dust the cinnamon over the top, and serve.

¾ cup (175 ml) brewed coffee

1 tablespoon (15 ml) sugar-free chocolate coffee flavoring syrup

1 or 2 drops orange extract

YIELD: 1 serving

4 calories; 0 g fat; trace protein; 1 g carbohydrate; 0 g dietary fiber per serving

CHOCOLATE-ORANGE COFFEE

I came up with this one morning when my husband was out of cream for his coffee. It kept me from having to run out to the store before breakfast, and he loved it!

Pour the coffee and stir in the syrup and the extract. That's all!

¾ cup (175 ml) brewed coffee

¼ cup (60 ml) heavy cream

24 drops liquid stevia (English toffee)

Pinch of ground cinnamon

Pinch of ground cloves

YIELD: 2 servings
107 calories; 11 g fat; 1 g protein; 2 g carbohydrate; trace dietary fiber per serving

SORT-OF-MEXICAN COFFEE

English toffee stevia stands in here for *piloncillo*, traditional Mexican brown sugar. Cross-cultural, no?

Stir together the coffee, cream, and liquid stevia. Pour into cups, and sprinkle a teeny bit of the spices over each cup before serving.

1½ quarts (1.5 L) water, plus more as needed

4 (family-size) tea bags

1 teaspoon liquid stevia (plain or lemon drop)*

---

*Alternative Sweeteners

  ½ teaspoon EZ-Sweetz Family Size

  ¼ teaspoon EZ-Sweetz Travel Size

YIELD: 16 servings, 1 cup (235 ml) each, or 1 gallon (3.8 L)
0 calories; 0 g fat; 0 g protein; 0 g carbohydrate; 0 g dietary fiber per serving

SWEET TEA

Sweet tea—iced tea with plenty of sugar in it—is the default summer beverage in the South. Here are the proportions for making a big pitcher of this classic without the sugar.

Bring the 1½ quarts (1.5 L) of water to a boil in a saucepan, then add the tea bags. Let it simmer for just a minute, then remove the pan from the heat and let it sit for about 10 minutes. Remove the tea bags, squeezing them out in the process.

Add the liquid stevia, and stir briefly to dissolve. Now pour this concentrate into a 1-gallon (3.8 L) pitcher, and add more water to fill. Serve over ice.

4 plain tea bags

4 Celestial Seasonings Raspberry Zinger herbal tea bags

1 quart (950 ml) boiling water

¼ cup (60 ml) lemon juice

¼ teaspoon liquid stevia (plain or lemon drop)*

1 bottle (1 L) sparkling water, raspberry flavor, unsweetened

*Alternative Sweeteners

12 drops EZ-Sweetz Family Size

6 drops EZ-Sweetz Travel Size

YIELD: 8 servings, about 1 cup (235 ml) each, or about 2 quarts (2 L)

5 calories; 0 g fat; trace protein; 1 g carbohydrate; trace dietary fiber per serving

SPARKLING RASPBERRY TEA

Light and refreshing! To change it up, try different flavors of sparkling water.

Put both kinds of tea bags in a heatproof pitcher, and pour the boiling water over them. Let them steep until cool. Using clean hands, squeeze the tea bags dry, and discard.

Add the lemon juice. Then start stirring the tea with a whisk before you start sprinkling the liquid stevia on the surface. Whisk it in gradually.

For each serving, pour ½ cup (120 ml) of the tea and about ½ cup (120 ml) chilled raspberry sparkling water into an ice-filled glass.

1 cup (235 ml) lemon juice

½ teaspoon liquid stevia (lemon drop or plain)*

Water, as needed

*Alternative Sweeteners

¼ teaspoon EZ-Sweetz Family Size

12 drops EZ-Sweetz Travel Size

YIELD: 8 servings, 1 cup (235 ml) each, or 2 quarts (2 L)

8 calories; 0 g fat; trace protein; 3 g carbohydrate; trace dietary fiber per serving

LEMONADE

You know—lemonade, but without the sugar. Fresh lemon juice is best, but bottled works fine. With this lemonade at 3 grams of carbohydrate per glass, you'll need to consider this a snack, and stick to just one serving.

Simple—just put everything in a 2-quart (2 L) pitcher and stir it up. Fill with water, and stir again. Serve over ice.

1½ cups (45 g)

dried hibiscus flowers

1½ quarts (1.5 L) boiling water

1 cup (235 ml) water, plus
more as needed

½ teaspoon liquid stevia
(plain or lemon drop)*

*Alternative Sweeteners

¼ teaspoon EZ-Sweetz
Family Size

12 drops EZ-Sweetz
Travel Size

YIELD: 6 servings, 1⅓ cups
(315 ml) each, or 2 quarts (2 L)
6 calories; trace fat; trace protein;
2 g carbohydrate; trace dietary
fiber per serving

1½ cups (45 g) hibiscus flowers

⅓ cup (40 g) lemon balm

⅓ cup (40 g) passionflower

3 tablespoons stevia herb,
or to taste*

2 tablespoons dried orange peel

*Alternative Sweeteners

It's hard to come up with
equivalencies for whole dried
stevia herb. If you'd like to use
another sweetener, simply
brew and chill, then sweeten
to taste with EZ-Sweetz or
liquid stevia.

YIELD: 8 servings
1 calorie; trace fat; trace protein;
trace carbohydrate; trace dietary
fiber per serving

HIBISCUS TEA

I first had hibiscus tea in Cozumel on the Low-Carb Cruise—I've gone on the cruise for years; it's where I got to know Dr. Westman and Jackie Eberstein, along with many other low-carb doctors, researchers, and dietitians, not to mention hundreds of wonderful people in the low-carb community. The sweet-tart fruity flavor and brilliant red color of hibiscus charmed me immediately. It has become a staple in my kitchen.

Super-simple: Put the hibiscus flowers in a heatproof pitcher, and pour in the boiling water. Let it sit till cool.

Strain your tea through a fine-mesh sieve, pressing all the liquid out of the flowers so as not to lose any. Pour a cup more water through them to get all the goodness and press again.

Pour into a 2-quart (2 L) pitcher, add water to fill, and stir in the stevia. Chill it well before serving.

RUBY RELAXER

This delicious, fruit punch–like herbal tea has become my go-to beverage on evenings when I don't care to drink alcohol. The lemon balm and passionflower are both mildly sedative, while the hibiscus, with its brilliant color, adds antioxidants. Herbs are cheapest purchased in bulk. If you have a local health food store that carries bulk herbs, try there. I usually buy online, at Mountain Rose Herbs.

Put all the herbs in a 2-quart (2 L) pitcher, and pour boiling water over them to fill. Let the tea stand and brew till cool.

Strain the tea through a fine-mesh sieve, pressing all you can out of the herbs, then pour a little more water through the herbs to rinse all the good out of them. Put the tea back in the pitcher, and add water to fill. (Remember, some of the space in the pitcher during brewing will have been taken up by the herbs.) Chill the tea.

This makes a concentrate. I like to mix it about 50/50 with cold water or cold sparkling water, but dilute to taste.

¼ cup (60 ml) heavy cream

1 can (12 ounces, or 355 ml) sugar-free soda, flavor of your choice, well chilled

---

YIELD: 1 serving

205 calories; 22 g fat; 1 g protein; 2 g carbohydrate; 0 g dietary fiber per serving

FARMER'S SODA

Reminiscent of an ice cream float, this makes a great summer dessert. Try it with sugar-free root beer, for a treat similar to a root beer float, or with orange soda if you miss sherbet. For a wider variety of flavors, use 1 fluid ounce (28 ml) of sugar-free coffee flavoring syrup, and fill with chilled club soda. This is infinitely variable—how about chocolate syrup and raspberry sparkling water? Vanilla syrup and lemon sparkling water? Caramel syrup and coconut sparkling water? Peach-flavored syrup and peach or pear sparkling water?

Simply pour the cream into the bottom of a large glass, and pour the soda over it.

CHAPTER 16
Desserts

Ideally, you'll be eating three meals per day, each with 5 grams or fewer of carbohydrate. Yet you're permitted a total of 20 grams. So where do the other 5 grams come from?

Guess what? They can come from dessert, if you like. You will find here a broad variety of desserts, some super-simple, some to satisfy your inner baker. Because they're nutritious, some can even serve as a quick breakfast.

A word of warning: Keep a sharp eye on portions. If you have a problem with sweets, you may do best to skip these recipes at the start. Or you can divide them up into portions, and refrigerate or freeze them that way, so you only take out one serving at a time. When my sister Kim was a little girl, and she was tempted by something she knew was off-limits, she'd say, "Put it in a high place, Mommy." Food that is not in your line of sight is less likely to speak to you.

1½ cups (150 g) walnuts

Boiling water, as needed

½ teaspoon vanilla extract

1 tablespoon (15 g) erythritol

Coconut oil, for frying

YIELD: 6 servings

191 calories; 18 g fat; 8 g protein;
4 g carbohydrate; 2 g dietary fiber
per serving

GLAZED WALNUTS

These make a nice little nibble after dinner, and are perfect with a cup of coffee. Take care when frying these—it's a quick jump from done to burnt.

Put your walnuts in a bowl, and cover with boiling water. Let them sit for just 4 or 5 minutes, then drain well.

Add the vanilla, and toss till it's evenly distributed. Add the erythritol, and toss until they're all evenly coated. Now spread your walnuts on a plate, and let them dry for an hour or two. This will minimize spitting when you fry them.

Put your big, heavy skillet over medium heat, and add ¼ inch (6 mm) of coconut oil. Let it get hot, then fry your walnuts a handful at a time, till just crisp. Cool, and store in a tightly lidded container.

---

2 tablespoons (28 g) butter

1 cup (100 g) shelled walnuts, pecans, or a combination of the two (I like the combo)

1½ to 2 tablespoons (22 to 30 g) erythritol

½ teaspoon ground cinnamon

YIELD: 4 servings (or possibly 5; remember, this is just a nibble)

239 calories; 24 g fat; 5 g protein;
5 g carbohydrate; 2 g dietary fiber
per serving

CINNAMON NUTS

Yummy! Butter-nut-cinnamon goodness. If you have any people with diabetes on your holiday gift list, tins of these make a nice present.

Melt the butter in a heavy skillet over medium heat, then add the nuts. Cook for 5 to 6 minutes, stirring from time to time. Then turn off the heat, and *immediately* sprinkle the erythritol and cinnamon over the top, and stir to distribute. (If you wait for the nuts to cool, the sweetener doesn't stick nearly as well.) I like these best warm, although they're quite nice when cooled.

CHEESECAKES

I have published a lot of cheesecake recipes, and with good reason: Cheesecake is wildly popular, endlessly variable, and—and this is important—"de-carbs" beautifully. Because the texture of cheesecake comes from protein and fat instead of from sugar, removing the sugar doesn't hurt the final product a bit—as you will see.

Another bonus: These cheesecakes are filling enough that a slice can stand in for breakfast. How's that for an eye-opener?!

2 pounds (900 g) cream cheese, at room temperature

2 cups (50 g) Splenda*

3 tablespoons (45 ml) heavy cream

5 eggs

---

*Alternative Sweeteners

2 cups (96 g) Stevia in the Raw

2 teaspoons liquid stevia (you could play with flavors)

2 teaspoons EZ-Sweetz Family Size

1 teaspoon EZ-Sweetz Travel Size

YIELD: 10 servings

365 calories; 36 g fat; 10 g protein; 3 g carbohydrate; 0 g dietary fiber per serving

THE MOST WONDERFUL CHEESECAKE

This recipe was named by the reader who contributed it for *500 More Low-Carb Recipes*. For a great add-on, pour a tablespoon (15 ml) or so of your favorite flavor of sugar-free coffee flavoring syrup over your slice of cheesecake.

Preheat oven to 375°F (190°C, or gas mark 5).

Mix everything together thoroughly with an electric mixer. Spread in a buttered 9-inch (23 cm) springform pan.

Bake the cheesecake for 10 minutes. Reduce the heat to 250°F (120°C) and bake for an additional hour.

At the end of the hour, remove the cake and run a knife around the edge of the pan.

Return the cake to the warm oven and let it sit until the oven cools (approximately another hour).

Chill in the fridge overnight and enjoy!

FOR MUFFINS:

5 eggs

16 ounces (450 g) full-fat ricotta

8 ounces (225 g) cream cheese, softened

1 cup (25 g) Splenda*

1 teaspoon almond extract

½ teaspoon vanilla extract

1½ tablespoons (8 g) unsweetened cocoa powder

FOR TOPPING:

½ cup (115 g) sour cream

1 tablespoon (1.5 g) Splenda*

¼ teaspoon vanilla extract

---

*Alternative Sweeteners

For muffins:

½ cup (120 g) erythritol *and* ½ teaspoon liquid stevia (plain or vanilla)

1 cup (48 g) Stevia in the Raw

½ teaspoon EZ-Sweetz Family Size

¼ teaspoon EZ-Sweetz Travel Size

For topping:

1 tablespoon (3 g) Stevia in the Raw

18 drops liquid stevia (vanilla)

YIELD: 12 servings
182 calories; 15 g fat; 8 g protein; 3 g carbohydrate; trace dietary fiber per serving

MARBLED CHEESECAKE MUFFINS

Linda Guiffre, who donated this recipe for *500 More Low-Carb Recipes*, says: "I drive a lot for my job so I'm particularly interested in portable food. These muffins are very quick and easy, and are pretty enough for company. They're also delicious and make a great snack or breakfast on the go."

Preheat oven to 350ºF (180ºC, or gas mark 4).

To make the muffins, in a medium bowl with an electric mixer, beat the eggs briefly until blended. Add the rest of the muffin ingredients, except the cocoa, to the bowl, and beat until completely blended.

Pour into muffin pans lined with cupcake liners (you'll need 12 liners) until about one-fifth of the batter remains in the bowl. Add the cocoa powder to the remaining batter (there is no need to worry about or be exact with amount of batter left over in the bowl; this recipe is very forgiving). Mix it in.

Slowly pour a dollop of the cocoa batter into the center of each cupcake so that you have a two-toned design. Bake for 30 to 35 minutes until the top is puffy and slightly cracked, and a toothpick inserted into the center comes out relatively clean. Remove the cupcakes from the oven to cool for a few minutes.

To make the topping, while the cupcakes are cooling, mix the topping ingredients together. Drop a rounded teaspoon of the topping onto the center of each cupcake (no need to flatten or shape) and return to the oven for another 5 minutes.

Cool and keep refrigerated. These freeze wonderfully, so you can always have some on hand.

VARIATION: Marbled Cheesecake

Linda adds: "For an impressive dessert presentation I make this cheesecake in a 7-inch [18 cm] springform pan, pouring the cocoa batter in a concentric design. I increase the topping to ¾ cup [172 g] sour cream, 1½ tablespoons [2.25 g] Splenda, and ⅓ teaspoon vanilla extract and spread it over the cheesecake. It's beautiful when sliced and gives the impression of being very labor-intensive—only you will know differently."

8 ounces (225 g) cream cheese, chilled

1 package (0.3 ounce, or 8.5 g) sugar-free gelatin, any flavor

---

YIELD: 8 servings

103 calories; 10 g fat; 3 g protein; 1 g carbohydrate; 0 g dietary fiber per serving

CREAM CHEESE BALLS

This idea has been going around the Internet to great reviews. It's so easy and simple, I had to pass it on. Bonus: The brightly colored balls are so pretty, a mixed plate of them would be nice to offer to company.

Cut your bar of cream cheese into 16 equal chunks. Use clean hands to roll each into a ball.

Pour the gelatin onto a plate, and roll each ball in the powder to coat. That's it.

Store these in an airtight container in the fridge.

2 tablespoons (28 ml) cold water

1 tablespoon (7 g) unflavored gelatin

¼ cup (60 ml) lemon juice

4 egg whites

¼ teaspoon cream of tartar

8 ounces (230 g) cream cheese

¼ teaspoon liquid stevia* (lemon drop), or more to taste

1 egg

½ cup (115 g) sour cream

1 teaspoon grated lemon zest

---

*Alternative Sweeteners

¼ cup (6 g) Splenda or (12 g) Stevia in the Raw

12 drops EZ-Sweetz Family Size

6 drops EZ-Sweets Travel Size

YIELD: 8 servings

156 calories; 13 g fat; 5 g protein; 4 g carbohydrate; trace dietary fiber per serving

LEMON-CHEESE MOUSSE

Like a light-and-fluffy cheesecake in a cup. If raw eggs worry you, look for pasteurized eggs.

First put the water in a small cup, and sprinkle the gelatin on top to soften. Let that sit for 10 minutes.

Meanwhile, put your lemon juice it in a small, nonreactive saucepan over low heat, and warm it up. When the gelatin is softened, add it to the lemon juice, and stir until the gelatin is completely dissolved and there are no granules left.

Now you need to beat your egg whites. Make sure the bowl and the beaters are completely grease-free, and that there's not even a tiny speck of yolk in your egg whites, or they won't whip! Beat them until they're frothy, then add the cream of tartar, and beat until stiff peaks form. Set aside for a minute or two while you do the next step.

In a mixing bowl, use your electric mixer to beat the cream cheese with the stevia and egg until it's light and fluffy. Now beat in the sour cream, lemon zest, and the gelatin mixture.

Gently fold this cream cheese mixture into the egg whites. Now pour the mousse into 8 pretty dessert dishes, and chill for at least 4 to 6 hours before serving.

2 cups (475 ml) heavy cream

⅓ cup (80 g) erythritol*

1 teaspoon vanilla extract

½ teaspoon liquid stevia*
(vanilla)

6 eggs

Pinch of salt

Pinch of ground nutmeg

8 tablespoons (120 ml)
sugar-free caramel coffee
flavoring syrup

---

*Alternative Sweeteners

To replace both the erythritol
and the liquid stevia:

¾ cup (18 g) Splenda or (36 g)
Stevia in the Raw

⅓ teaspoon EZ-Sweetz
Family Size

18 drops EZ-Sweetz Travel
Size

(When making any of these
substitutions, add an extra
¼ teaspoon vanilla extract.)

To replace only the liquid
stevia:

½ cup (12 g) Splenda or
(24 g) Stevia in the Raw

¼ teaspoon EZ Sweets
Family Size

12 drops EZ-Sweetz Travel
Size

YIELD: 8 servings
256 calories; 25 g fat; 5 g protein;
2 g carbohydrate; trace dietary
fiber per serving

FLAN

I adore baked custard, and this one is rich and silky. It's a great dessert, but consider this for breakfast as well.

Preheat oven to 350ºF (180ºC, or gas mark 4). Grease a 10-inch (25 cm) pie plate or a 9½-inch (24 cm) deep-dish pie plate.

Put the cream, erythritol, vanilla, stevia, eggs, salt, and nutmeg in your blender, and run till it's all well combined.

Put a shallow baking pan on the oven rack. Place the prepared pie plate in it. Pour water in the outer pan up to within about ½ inch (1 cm) of the rim of the pie plate. Now pour the custard mixture into the pie plate.

Bake for 50 to 60 minutes, or until just set.

Carefully remove the pie plate from the water bath to let it cool for 30 minutes before chilling.

You can run a knife around the edge and invert the flan onto a plate, then top with the caramel syrup to serve, but it's easier to just cut wedges like a pie, or spoon it out. Still top it with the syrup to serve!

2 cups (270 g) hazelnuts

1 cup (128 g) vanilla whey protein powder

½ teaspoon salt

¼ teaspoon baking powder

1 cup (225 g) butter, at room temperature

½ cup (120 g) powdered erythritol*

1 egg

2 tablespoons (28 ml) water

---

*Alternative Sweeteners

½ cup (12 g) Splenda or (24 g) Stevia in the Raw

YIELD: 48 servings (1 cookie)
91 calories; 8 g fat; 5 g protein; 1 g carbohydrate; trace dietary fiber per serving

HAZELNUT SHORTBREAD

Love Walkers Shortbread cookies? You have to try these!

Preheat oven to 325°F (170°C, or gas mark 3).

First grind the hazelnuts to a fine meal in a food processor. Add the vanilla whey protein, salt, and baking powder, and pulse to combine.

Using an electric mixer, beat the butter until it's fluffy. Add the erythritol and beat well again. Next beat in the egg, again combining well. Now beat in the hazelnut mixture, in 3 or 4 additions. Finally, beat in the water.

You will now have a soft, sticky dough. Line a shallow baking pan—a jelly roll pan is best; mine is 11½ × 15½ inches (29 × 39 cm)—with baking parchment, and turn the dough out onto the parchment. Cover it with another piece of parchment, and through the top sheet, press the dough out into an even layer covering the whole pan. It should be about ¼ inch (6 mm) thick. Peel off the top sheet of parchment, and use a knife with a nonserrated, thin blade to score the dough into squares. Bake for 25 to 30 minutes, or until golden. You'll need to re-score the lines before removing the shortbread from the pan—use a straight up-and-down motion and the shortbread will be less likely to break.

⅔ cup (85 g) vanilla whey protein powder

⅔ cup (75 g) almond meal

1 teaspoon xanthan or guar

½ cup (112 g) butter, at room temperature

½ cup (109 g) coconut oil—solid, not melted—but not chilled and rock hard

¼ cup (60 g) powdered erythritol, plus extra for dusting

½ teaspoon salt

1 egg yolk

1⅓ cups (105 g) shredded coconut meat (unsweetened, not Angel Flake)

YIELD: 48 servings (1 cookie)
66 calories; 6 g fat; 3 g protein; 1 g carbohydrate; trace dietary fiber per serving

MERRY CRISPNESS SHORTBREAD

Rich and tender, and sheer heaven with a cup of tea. As the name suggests, I created these as a Christmas cookie.

Preheat oven to 325ºF (170ºC, or gas mark 3). Line a jelly roll pan with baking parchment.

In a bowl, whisk together the protein powder, almond meal, and xanthan so they're evenly distributed.

In another bowl, using your electric mixer, beat the butter and coconut oil together until they're fluffy and creamy

Beat in the erythritol and salt, mixing till it's completely blended—scrape down the sides of the bowl as needed. Now beat in the egg yolk.

Beat in the almond meal mixture in 3 additions, making sure each is well blended before adding more. Finally, beat in the shredded coconut.

Turn the dough out onto the parchment-lined jelly roll pan. Place another sheet of parchment over it, and using a rolling pin and your hands, press the dough out into an even sheet, completely covering the pan—I did need to use my hands to get it all the way into the corners, nipping off bits of dough where there was a bit too much and adding it where it was needed.

When you have a beautiful rectangle of dough, peel off the top parchment and use a thin, straight-bladed knife to score it into squares.

Bake for 10 to 12 minutes, until golden. Keep an eye on it—it goes from golden to overbrowned quickly.

When your shortbread comes out of the oven, re-score it, then use a sifter to dust it with a little more erythritol—I used 2 to 3 tablespoons (30 to 45 g).

Let your shortbread cool in the pan, then use a pancake turner to transfer to an airtight container or cookie tin.

12 ounces (340 g) walnuts

½ cup (120 g) erythritol, divided

4 eggs

Pinch of cream of tartar

⅓ teaspoon EZ-Sweetz Family Size*

2 teaspoons lemon zest

Pinch of salt

2 tablespoons (30 g) powdered erythritol*, for topping

---

*Alternative Sweeteners

Do not replace the ½ cup (120 g) erythritol.

You can replace the EZ-Sweetz Family Size with:

18 drops EZ-Sweetz Travel Size

2 tablespoons (3 g) Splenda or (6 g) Stevia in the Raw to sprinkle on top

---

YIELD: 12 servings
195 calories; 18 g fat; 9 g protein; 4 g carbohydrate; 1 g dietary fiber per serving

ITALIAN WALNUT CAKE

This traditional Italian cake is a clear demonstration that a few simple ingredients, properly combined, can yield extraordinary results. If it takes you a few days to eat up all of your Italian Walnut Cake—which it will, unless the family is helping—the sweetener on top will melt, leaving a glazed look instead of powdery whiteness, but it will still taste wonderful. This would be fabulous with a simple cup of espresso.

Preheat oven to 350ºF (180ºC, or gas mark 4). Coat a 9-inch (23 cm) spring-form pan with nonstick cooking spray, and line the bottom with a circle of baking parchment, or a reusable nonstick pan liner.

Put the walnuts in your food processor with the S-blade in place. Pulse till the nuts are chopped medium-fine. Add 2 tablespoons (30 g) of the erythritol, and pulse until the nuts are finely ground, but not oily. (Don't overprocess. You don't want nut butter!)

Separate your eggs. Since even the tiniest speck of egg yolk will cause the whites to stubbornly refuse to whip, do yourself a big favor and separate each one into a small dish or cup before adding the white to the bowl you plan to whip them in! Then, if you break a yolk, you've only messed up that white. (Give that one to the dog, or save it for scrambled eggs for breakfast.) Put the whites in a deep, narrow mixing bowl, and put the yolks in a larger mixing bowl.

Add the pinch of cream of tartar to the whites, and using your electric mixer (not a blender or food processor), whip the egg whites until they stand in stiff peaks. Set aside.

In a larger bowl, beat the yolks with the remaining 6 tablespoons (90 g) erythritol, and all of the EZ-Sweetz, until the mixture is pale yellow and very creamy—at least 3 to 4 minutes. Beat in the lemon zest and the salt.

Stir the ground walnuts into the yolk mixture—you can use the electric mixer, but the mixture will be so thick, I think a spoon is easier. When that's well combined, gently fold in the egg whites one-third at a time, using a rubber scraper. Incorporate each third well before adding the next third. When all the egg whites are folded in, gently pour the batter into the prepared pan.

Bake for 45 minutes. Sprinkle the top with the 2 tablespoons (30 g) powdered erythritol while the cake is hot, then let cool before serving. Cut into thin wedges to serve.

2 pounds (900 g) cream cheese, at room temperature

1 cup (245 g) canned pumpkin puree (not pumpkin pie filling)

3 tablespoons (45 ml) heavy cream

1 teaspoon EZ-Sweetz Family Size*

1 teaspoon ground cinnamon

1 teaspoon ground ginger

½ teaspoon ground nutmeg

5 eggs

---

*Alternative Sweeteners

1 teaspoon EZ-Sweetz Travel Size

2 teaspoons liquid stevia (English toffee or plain)

YIELD: 10 servings

375 calories; 36 g fat; 10 g protein; 5 g carbohydrate; 1 g dietary fiber per serving

(NS) THE MOST WONDERFUL PUMPKIN CHEESECAKE

Wondering what you're serving for Thanksgiving dessert? We've got you covered. If you'd like to call this 12 servings, you could afford to sprinkle a few chopped Cinnamon Nuts (page 171) over your slice for textural contrast. Just sayin'.

Preheat oven to 375ºF (190ºC, or gas mark 5). Line a 9-inch (23 cm) springform pan with nonstick foil, covering the seam at the bottom. Butter the whole thing well, bottom and sides, or coat with nonstick cooking spray.

Simply put all your ingredients in a big mixing bowl, and beat with an electric mixer until it's all smoothly blended. Pour into the prepared pan. Place in the oven. Put a roasting pan with 1 inch (2.5 cm) of water in the oven on the rack beneath.

Bake the cheesecake for 10 minutes. Reduce the heat to 250ºF (120ºC) and bake for an additional hour.

At the end of the hour, remove the cake and run a knife around the edge of the pan.

Return the cheesecake to the warm oven and let it sit until the oven cools (approximately another hour).

Chill in the fridge overnight and enjoy!

(NS)

1 package (0.3 ounces, or 8.5 g) sugar-free raspberry gelatin

1 cup (235 ml) boiling water

2 teaspoons lemon juice

Grated zest of ½ orange (feed the orange to the kids)

¾ cup (115 g) frozen blackberries, partly thawed

1 cup (235 ml) heavy cream, divided

12 drops liquid stevia (vanilla)*

_____

*Alternative Sweeteners
   Use a drop or two of liquid Splenda plus ½ teaspoon vanilla extract in the whipped cream.

_____

YIELD: 6 servings
156 calories; 15 g fat; 1 g protein; 5 g carbohydrate; 1 g dietary fiber per serving

MIXED BERRY CUPS

For you raspberry and blackberry lovers. If you have glass dessert dishes, use them! The pretty color will show.

Put the gelatin, water, lemon juice, and orange zest in a blender, and whirl for 10 to 15 seconds to dissolve the gelatin. Add the blackberries, and whirl again, just long enough to blend in the berries.

   Put the blender container in the refrigerator for 10 minutes—just until the mixture is starting to thicken a bit.

   Add ¾ cup (175 ml) of the heavy cream, and run the blender just long enough to mix it all in—about 10 to 15 seconds. Pour into 6 pretty little dessert cups and chill. Whip the remaining ¼ cup (60 ml) cream with the vanilla liquid stevia, and dollop a spoonful on each serving for garnish.

2 ounces (56 g) unsweetened baking chocolate

1 cup (225 g) butter

½ cup (120 g) erythritol

½ cup (12 g) Splenda*

2 eggs

½ cup (64 g) vanilla whey protein powder

Pinch of salt

_____

*Alternative Sweeteners
   Replace the Splenda with ½ teaspoon liquid stevia (chocolate)

_____

YIELD: 12 servings
208 calories; 19 g fat; 9 g protein; 2 g carbohydrate; 1 g dietary fiber per serving

DANA'S BROWNIES

Yes, brownies. Furthermore, these have a low enough carb count that you could have them in addition to a super-low-carb supper.

Preheat oven to 350ºF (180ºC, or gas mark 4). Coat an 8-inch (20 cm) square baking pan with nonstick cooking spray.

   In the top of a double boiler, or in a saucepan over a heat diffuser, set on lowest possible heat, melt the chocolate and butter together. Stir until they're well combined. Scrape this into a mixing bowl.

   Add the erythritol, and stir well, then stir in the Splenda. Next, beat in the eggs, one at a time. Stir in the protein powder and salt.

   Pour into the prepared pan and bake for 15 to 20 minutes. Do not overbake! Cut into 12 squares, and let cool in the pan. Store in an airtight container in the refrigerator.

BIBLIOGRAPHY

WEBSITES

American Diabetes Association
www.diabetes.org
American Podiatric Medical Association: Diabetic Wound Care
www.apma.org
Centers for Disease Control and Prevention
www.cdc.gov
Cureality Blog
www.cureality.com/blog (post on 6/6/10)
Diabetes Teaching Center at the University of California, San Francisco: Diabetes Education Online
http://dtc.ucsf.edu
Diapedia.org: The Living Textbook of Diabetes
www.diapedia.org
Dietary Guidelines for Americans 2010
www.dietaryguidelines.gov
Food Insight
www.foodinsight.org
Joslin Diabetes Center
www.joslin.org
National Academy on an Aging Society
www.agingsociety.org
National Institute of Health: National Institute of Diabetes and Digestive and Kidney Diseases
www.niddk.nih.gov
National Institutes of Health: National Eye Institute
www.nei.nih.gov
USDA National Nutrient Database for Standard Reference
https://ndb.nal.usda.gov
U.S. Department of Commerce: National Technical Information Service
http://ageconsearch.umn.edu/bitstream/154874/2/sb915.pdf

PUBLICATIONS

Bazzano, L., Hu, T., Reynolds, K., et al. "Effects of Low Carbohydrate and Low-Fat Diets: A Randomized Trial," *Annals of Internal Medicine*, 161(5): 309–18.
Fine, E., Segal-Isaacson, C.J., Feinman, R., et al. "Targeting insulin inhibition as a metabolic therapy in advanced cancer: A pilot safety and feasibility dietary trial in 10 patients," *Nutrition*, 28(10): 1028–35.

Friedmann, A., Chambers, M., Kamendulis, L., et al. "Short-Term Changes after a Weight Reduction Intervention in Advanced Diabetic Nephropathy," *Journal of the American Society of Nephrology*, 8(11): 1892–8.
Hellerstein, MK. "Carbohydrate-induced hypertriglyceridemia: modifying factors and implications for cardiovascular risk," *Current Opinion in Lipidology*, 13(1): 33–40.
Kekwick, A. , Pawan, G.L. "Calorie Intake in Relation to Body-Weight Changes in the Obese," *The Lancet*, July 28, 1956.
Mavropoulos, J., Yancy, W., Hepburn, J. et al. "The effects of a low-carbohydrate, ketogenic diet on the polycystic ovary syndrome: A pilot study," *Nutrition and Metabolism*, 2005(2): 35.
Paoli, A., Bianco, A., Damiani, E., et al. "Ketogenic Diet in Neuromuscular and Neurodegenerative Diseases," *BioMed Research International*, 2014: 474296.
Poplawski MM., Mastaitis JW., Isoda F., et al. "Reversal of Diabetic Nephropathy by a Ketogenic Diet," PLoS ONE 6(4): e18604. doi:10.1371/journal.pone.0018604
Young, C., Scanlan, S., Hae Sook, I., Lutwak, L. "Effect on body composition and other parameters in obese young men of carbohydrate level of reduction diet," *The American Journal of Clinical Nutrition*, 24(3): 290–6.
Sondike, SB., Copperman N., Jacobson, MS. "Effects of a low-carbohydrate diet on weight loss and cardiovascular risk factor in overweight adolescents," *Journal of Pediatrics*, 142(3):253–8.
Tiwari, S., Riazi, S., Ecelbarger, CA. "Insulin's impact on renal sodium transport and blood pressure in health, obesity, and diabetes," *The American Journal of Physiology: Renal*, 293(4): F974–84.
Walsh, Bryan. "Fnding the War on Fat," *Time* magazine, June 12, 2014.
Zechner, R., Kiensberger, PC., Haemmerle, G., Zimmermann, R. "Adipose triglyceride lipase and the lipolytic catabolism of cellular fat stores," *Journal of Lipid Research*, 50(1): 3–21.

BOOK

Eades, Michael and Eades, Mary Dan. *Protein Power: The High-Protein/Low Carbohydrate Way to Lose Weight, Feel Fit, and Boost Your Health-in Just Weeks!* (New York: Bantam Books: 1996)

ABOUT THE AUTHOR

In retrospect, Dana Carpender's career seems inevitable: She's been cooking since she had to stand on a step stool to reach the stove. She was also a dangerously sugar-addicted child, eventually stealing from her parents to support her habit, and was in Weight Watchers by age eleven. At nineteen, Dana read her first book on nutrition, and she recognized herself in a list of symptoms of reactive hypoglycemia. She ditched sugar and white flour and was dazzled by the near instantaneous improvement in her physical and mental health. A lifetime nutrition buff was born.

Unfortunately, in the late 1980s and early 1990s, Dana got sucked into the low-fat/high-carb mania, and whole-grain-and-beaned her way up to a size 20, with nasty energy swings, constant hunger, and borderline high blood pressure. In 1995, she read a nutrition book from the 1950s that stated that obesity had nothing to do with how much one ate, but was rather a carbohydrate intolerance disease. She thought, "What the heck, might as well give it a try." Three days later, her clothes were loose, her hunger was gone, and her energy level was through the roof. She never looked back, and she has now been low-carb for twenty years and counting—more than one-third of her life.

Realizing that this change was permanent, and being a cook at heart, Dana set about creating as varied and satisfying a cuisine as she could with a minimal carb load. And being an enthusiastic, gregarious sort, she started sharing her experience. By 1997, she was writing about it. The upshot is more than 2,500 recipes published and more than a million books sold—and she still has ideas left to try! Dana lives in Bloomington, Indiana, with her husband, three dogs, and a cat, all of whom are well and healthily fed.

INDEX